Living Well
with an
Ostomy

Living Well
with an
Ostomy

Elizabeth Rayson

First published in Canada in 2003 by
Your Health Press™, a division of Sarahealth Inc.
In association with Trafford Publishing.

Printed in Victoria, Canada

National Library of Canada Cataloguing in Publication Data

Rayson, Elizabeth
    Living well with an ostomy / Elizabeth Rayson.
Includes bibliographical references and index.

ISBN 1-4120-0081-5

1. Nephrostomy—Popular works. 2. Enterostomy—Popular works.
3. Ostomates—Health and hygiene. I. Title.

RD540.R39 2003   617.5'5   C2003-901539-4

IMPORTANT NOTICE:

The purpose of this book is to educate. It is sold with the understanding that the author and publisher shall have neither liability nor responsibility for any injury caused or alleged to be caused directly or indirectly by the information contained in this book. While every effort has been made to ensure its accuracy, the book's contents should not be construed as medical advice. Each person's health needs are unique. To obtain recommendations appropriate to your particular situation, please consult a qualified health care provider. The herbal remedies recommended in this book are for education purposes only and should not be used without consulting a qualified expert in herbal medicine.

This book was published *on-demand* in cooperation with Trafford Publishing.
On-demand publishing is a unique process and service of making a book available for retail sale to the public taking advantage of on-demand manufacturing and Internet marketing. **On-demand publishing** includes promotions, retail sales, manufacturing, order fulfilment, accounting and collecting royalties on behalf of the author.

Suite 6E, 2333 Government St., Victoria, B.C. V8T 4P4, CANADA
Phone	250-383-6864	Toll-free	1-888-232-4444 (Canada & US)
Fax	250-383-6804	E-mail	sales@trafford.com
Web site	www.trafford.com	TRAFFORD PUBLISHING IS A DIVISION OF TRAFFORD HOLDINGS LTD.
Trafford Catalogue #03-0444		www.trafford.com/robots/03-0444.html	

10   9   8   7   6   5   4

OTHER YOUR HEALTH PRESS™ TITLES

Stopping Cancer At The Source by M. Sara Rosenthal, Ph.D. (2001)
Women and Unwanted Hair by M. Sara Rosenthal, Ph.D. (2001)
Living Well with Celiac Disease: Abundance Beyond Wheat and Gluten by Claudine Crangle (2002)
The Thyroid Cancer Book by M. Sara Rosenthal, Ph.D. (2002)

Soon to be released...

Thyroid Eye Disease: Understanding Graves' Ophthalmopathy by Elaine Moore (2003)

Pediatric Glaucoma and Cataract Disease: Your Questions Answered by The Pediatric Glaucoma and Cataract Disease Foundation and edited by Alex Levin, M.D., F.R.C.P., Director, Ophthalmology, The Hospital for Sick Children (2003)

Premature Menopause: When the Change Comes Too Soon by Karin Banerd (2003)

Healing Injuries: Fractures, Broken Bones, Whiplash, Bursitis, Torn Muscles & Tendons & More by Michelle Cook (2003)

ACKNOWLEDGMENTS

I wish to thank the following groups and individuals whose expertise and support helped make the job of writing this book so much more pleasurable.

First, I'd like to thank all the individuals at the Ostomy Toronto group who offered their time and knowledge to help bring this book into being. I'd especially like to thank Candace Miron, Director, United Ostomy Association of Canada; Lorne Aronson, President, United Ostomy Association of Canada, and Carol Rodda, Ostomy Resource Centre Coordinator. I'd also like to thank the United Ostomy Association of Canada for their generous permission to use the ostomy diagrams from their publication, *Ostomy – A Reference Guide*. Furthermore, the guidance and expertise of the medical review team at the United Ostomy Association helped make this book a reality.

Gabriela A. Ghitulescu, M.D., Jewish General Hospital; Assistant Professor of Surgery, McGill University also provided a meticulous medical review, and was kind enough to write this book's foreword. Her help was invaluable.

And special thanks to Paula Krulicki of Colborne Communications, who handled the book's cover and text design, for all her hard work and expertise.

I'd also like to recognize all those at Your Health Press™ who encouraged me to take on this project. I'd especially like to thank Larissa Kostoff, my editor – without her generous support, expertise and feedback, this book would not have been written.

CONTENTS

Foreword 11

Introduction...13

Chapter 1:   Understanding ostomy 15
            Congenital conditions
            Injury
            Colorectal cancer
            Familial adenomatous polyposis (FAP)
            Inflammatory bowel disease

Chapter 2:   Types of ostomies 25
            Colostomy: the basics
            Ileostomy: the basics
            Urostomy: the basics

Chapter 3:   Before ostomy surgery...41
            Preparing for ostomy surgery
            Pre-surgery homeopathy and aromatherapy
            Pre-surgery procedures to expect
            Charter of Ostomate's Rights

Chapter 4:   After ostomy surgery...55
            In hospital and after
            Post-surgery homeopathy and aromatherapy
            Bladder infections
            Life goes on

Chapter 5:   Basic ostomy care 63
                 If it's my ostomy, why do I feel like it's managing me?
                 Options for managing colostomies
                 Options for managing ileostomies
                 Basic care for urostomies

Chapter 6:   Selecting an appliance 71
                 About appliances
                 Appliance accessories
                 Ostomy care Q & A

Chapter 7:   Diet, skin care and medication 79
                 Dietary guidelines and nutrition
                 Skin care
                 Medication

Chapter 8:   Working, playing, and seeing the world 97
                 Taking care of business: dealing with your ostomy
                   on the job
                 Ostomies and the sporting life
                 On the road with an ostomy
                 Travel tips for irrigation

Chapter 9:   Body image, relationships and sexuality 105
                 The grieving process
                 His and hers: how will your ostomy affect your sex life?
                 Women and their ostomies
                 What about pregnancy?
                 Men and their ostomies
                 Dos and don'ts for great sex

Chapter 10: Considerations for special groups 125
                 Ostomy care for the elderly
                 Babies and children with ostomies
                 Teenagers and ostomies
                 Issues related to ethnicity and culture

Final Word 139
Resources 141
Glossary 157
Bibliography 167

FOREWORD

Most people who are told they'll have a stoma must, at the same time, face the prospect of undergoing major surgery for a serious condition. It may seem that the stoma, in such cases, would be the least worrisome. But it's become clear to me that for most people the prospect of an ostomy is a major source of stress, simply because they don't know what to expect. Only by providing the facts about ostomy surgery and living with an ostomy to those who need them can we minimize this fear of the unknown.

This is precisely what this book does and as such I welcome it to the armamentarium of resources at the disposition of healthcare professionals. With it, we can help ease the fears of our patients, and improve their care.

Gabriela A. Ghitulescu, M.D.
Jewish General Hospital;
Assistant Professor of Surgery
McGill University

INTRODUCTION

If you have or will be getting an ostomy, this book is for you. The first part of the book covers basic information about the different types of ostomies, including the different surgical options available today. It also lets you know what to expect from ostomy surgery and provides advice on how to ease your recovery from ostomy surgery. Later chapters focus on some of the psycho/social issues that may surface as a result of ostomy surgery, including those unique to certain groups, such as children, young adults and seniors.

There are many good resources that focus on specific issues for people with ostomies, and I haven't tried to tell you "everything there is to know" in this book. I do hope, though, that *Living Well with an Ostomy* will give you enough information to make the most of life with an ostomy. And to help you find even more information, the Resources section at the back of the book contains a host of references to additional sources.

Don't feel obliged to read this book from front to back. I've tried to organize the book so that it lets you easily find what you're looking for. So use this book as your guide by picking and choosing the information most pertinent to you. Here are some tips on how to make the most of *Living Well with an Ostomy:*

- If you've just learned that you need an ostomy and you want to get a bit of background, read chapters 1 and 2 first to get a feel for just what an ostomy is. You can also turn straight to chapter 3 for information about preparing for ostomy surgery. Then, you may want to browse through the remaining chapters for more information about your particular situation.
- If you've had an ostomy for many years, take a look at the first two chapters to see if there's information there that you don't already

know. Then, focus on chapters that contain information more specific to your needs.

- If you have a child, partner or friend with an ostomy, turn to the chapter that addresses these groups. For example, chapter 9 looks at relationships and sexuality; chapter 10 goes into greater depth on those issues common to special groups like children and senior citizens.

And if from time to time you come across language you don't understand – don't worry! I've tried to anticipate this by providing detailed definitions in the Glossary on page 155. So, let's start by answering the question most central to this book: *What is an ostomy anyway?*

1
UNDERSTANDING OSTOMY

So what is an ostomy, anyway?

Ostomy surgery is a type of surgery that's needed by those who don't have normal bladder or bowel function because of disease (such as inflammatory bowel disease and colon cancer), congenital conditions or injury. An ostomy is an artificial opening between a cavity and the surface of the body. If you've been told you need an ostomy, you may have been experiencing repeated incontinence of stool or urine due to problems with bowel and bladder function. Your doctor may have diagnosed cancer of the digestive or urinary tracts, or you may have been suffering from an inflammatory bowel disease, such as colitis or Crohn's disease, for some time. Your doctor may have recommended an ostomy as a way to eliminate the disease so that you can regain your health.

During ostomy surgery, a new opening (called a stoma) is created in the abdominal wall. The body can then release waste through the stoma, and bypass exisiting problems in the bowel or bladder. Most people with ostomies wear appliances, or pouches, over the stoma, although some choose other methods of managing the stoma, such as irrigation. We'll be exploring all these ostomy care methods in later chapters of this book.

It's obvious that getting an ostomy is a life-changing experience. If you've been told that you need an ostomy, it's normal and natural for you to feel scared, unsure, anxious – and even angry that this terrible thing is happening to you.

There's no denying the fact that getting an ostomy will challenge you. You'll not only need to learn how to deal with the practical aspects of ostomy care, you'll also need to grapple with the changes to your body. How will you be able to live with a stoma? Will it prevent you from traveling? Dressing well? Playing sports? Eating the foods you love? Enjoying satisfying romantic and sexual relationships?

The good news is that managing successfully with your ostomy is well within your grasp. This book is designed to answer your questions, remove your fears and provide you with a roadmap to living well with your ostomy.

Although it may seem incredible now, there will come a time when you won't think twice about your ostomy. It'll become just another part of you. Sure, your ostomy requires that you learn some specialized skills, such as changing a pouch or irrigating a colostomy. It's not uncommon for people who are dealing with ostomy surgery to feel that they're changed forever – both inside and out. Some people may even feel that they've been disfigured or violated by ostomy surgery. But, ultimately, your ostomy is only a small part of the essential person that is you. And that essential person hasn't changed or become less active, adventurous, stylish or romantic just because she or he now has an ostomy. On the contrary, many people who've had ostomy surgery will tell you that their surgery marked the start of a new, more expansive phase in their lives.

June, 32, who had suffered from IBD for five years prior to surgery, tells this story:

> I was so sick with colitis that I couldn't wait for surgery – I even asked my doctor to call me if there were any cancellations. And even though it was uncomfortable, the surgery was definitely worth it. Yes, I was afraid, but I knew I couldn't let the fear stop me from getting well. When I went out for my first walk with my husband after surgery, it felt so good! There were birds singing, flowers blossoming, children laughing in the park… and I was finally enjoying being outside, which I hadn't been able to do when I was ill. I felt like I had an opportunity to start over again. I felt like I had been given a second chance at life.

A bit of background for the history buffs

Later in this chapter, we'll explore the different types of ostomies in more detail. But first, let's take quick look at the history of ostomy surgery.

Nineteenth century medical journals debated surgical techniques for ostomies, but it wasn't until later in the nineteenth century when ostomy surgery became more common, and surgical techniques improved, that patients began reaping the benefits. It's not that there weren't successes in early attempts at ostomy surgery. For example, there's the case of Miss Miriam Cooney. After undergoing ostomy surgery in 1884 at the age of 20, she celebrated her 104th birthday in 1968 – after 84 years of living with her colostomy! Not to mention the fact that she'd survived several brothers and sisters to get to this milestone.

If necessity is the mother of invention, then it was battle casualties that perfected some of the earliest ostomy surgeries. In 1707, for example, life-saving enterostomal surgery was successfully performed on injured soldiers in Flanders, France.

But disease, of course, also played a role. One eighteenth-century woman, 73-year-old Margaret White, had her abdominal wall break down. This allowed the bowel to prolapse ("fall out") from her pre-existing hernia. But White's doctor was able to remove the diseased bowel, and surgically draw the healthy bowel out to her abdomen. Margaret White lived for many years afterward.

Later in the nineteenth century, the loop colostomy was performed for the first time. From about that time until the present, the basic concepts underlying the surgical construction of an ostomy have remained the same – though many technical improvements have taken place. One of these is the development of the abdominoperineal (A-P) resection. First performed in 1908 by Dr. William Ernest Miles, this surgery is still the "gold standard" for many rectal cancers located near the anus.

And technical improvements continue to be developed. (Pouch devices, for example, have improved significantly since ostomies began to be performed.)Later in this chapter we'll explore options for ostomy surgery, such as the creation of a continent ileostomy. The viability of these options depends, however, on the type of injury or illness. For example, pelvic pouch surgery is sometimes an option for those with ulcerative colitis, but not for those who suffer from Crohn's disease. For Crohn's disease sufferers, an ileorectal anastomosis procedure can work well in many cases. Both these procedures offer an alternative to the conventional ostomy surgery, in which an external stoma is created and a pouch is worn to collect the body's waste.

Why get an ostomy?

Unlike most of the ostomy surgery performed in previous centuries, in the 21st century, it's unlikely (though by no means unheard of) for ostomy surgery to happen as a result of a war injury – at least in North America. Injury is one of the causes of ostomy surgery, but in North America the wounds are more likely to be inflicted during an automobile accident than in hand-to-hand combat. Today, most people get an ostomy as a result of severe complications from inflammatory bowel diseases, colorectal cancer, familial polyposis, congenital conditions or injury.

An informal 2002 poll of 630 members of the Evansville Chapter of the United Ostomy Association gives a general idea of what conditions most commonly justify the need for ostomy surgery. Respondents answered as follows when asked the question: *why did you get an ostomy or continent procedure* (more about these later)?

- Some type of cancer: 29 percent (183 respondents)
- Ulcerative colitis: 37 percent (233 respondents)
- Crohn's disease: 19 percent (119 respondents)
- Accident, injury or congenital condition: 6 percent (36 respondents)
- Familial adenomatous polyposis – FAP: 1 percent (5 respondents)
- Other: 8 percent (54 respondents)

So if you've been told you need an ostomy, you're probably suffering from one of these conditions. On the other hand, having colon cancer or inflammatory bowel disease doesn't necessarily mean that you will, inevitably, need an ostomy. The next section explains more about each of these conditions, and tells you how to tell when surgery is necessary in each case.

Congenital Conditions

Congenital (present at birth) conditions like spina bifida and Hirschsprung's disease may lead to ostomy surgery. In fact, congenital conditions are the reason most children have ostomies. In many cases, ostomies performed due to congenital conditions are temporary – intended to give the infant's body enough time to develop to the extent that the original problem can be surgically corrected.

Injury

It's also possible to require an ostomy as the result of trauma sustained during an accident (such as an automobile accident). Again, ostomy surgery may be performed as a temporary measure, to give injured tissue a chance to heal.

Colorectal Cancer

According to the American Gastroenterological Association (AGA), colorectal cancer is the second leading cause of death from cancer in the United States. The National Cancer Institute estimates that more than 65,000 people will die this year of colorectal cancer in the United States. Experts also estimate that more than 160,000 new cases of the disease will be diagnosed annually, and 80 to 90 million people are considered at risk because of age and/or other factors.

These are sobering facts, but there's good news, too. Colorectal cancer is actually one of the most treatable forms of cancer. With early diagnosis and proper treatment, many colorectal cancer survivors lead long and healthy lives.

The AGA lists several risk factors for colorectal cancer:

- Anyone over the age of 50 is considered to be at risk for developing colorectal cancer. Approximately 90 percent of colorectal cancers occur in people over the age of 50.
- Individuals with either a personal or a family history of colorectal cancer or polyps, or who have suffered from an inflammatory bowel disease, such as ulcerative colitis or Crohn's disease, are at higher risk for developing the disease.
- Women with a history of ovarian and uterine cancers have an increased risk of developing colorectal cancer.
- High-fat, low-fiber diets appear to be associated with colorectal cancer. Research also suggests that certain methods of cooking meats (such as frying, barbecuing and broiling) create high levels of heterocyclic amines (HCAs). HCAs are cancer-causing chemicals associated with the development of various types of cancer, including colorectal cancer.

Colorectal cancer is often difficult to diagnose. Some people have no symptoms – or, they may experience fatigue; abdominal cramping and bloating; diarrhea; constipation; blood-tinged stool; and unexplained weight loss. (Often there's a feeling that the bowel doesn't empty properly, and the stool may appear narrower than usual.)

Treating colorectal cancer

Treatment for colorectal cancer may include surgery, chemotherapy or radiation – or a combination of the three. Most people with colorectal cancer undergo surgery to remove the cancer, and prevent complications such as bleeding, obstruction, perforation, or spread of malignant cells. During surgery, the surgeon removes the unhealthy part of the colon and then reconnects the healthy parts. Among patients with more aggressive tumors, chemotherapy and/or radiotherapy are recommended to prevent or treat spread of malignant cells

It's the location of the tumor that will likely determine whether or not you will need a permanent ostomy. Tumors located further down in the gastrointestinal tract, on or very near the anus, are more difficult to surgically remove without also removing too much of the rectal tissue. Sometimes, it's just impossible for surgeons to remove enough of the tumor to preserve your health while also preserving your rectum. If your doctor suggests ostomy surgery for colorectal cancer, the resulting ostomy will likely be permanent if most or all of the rectum had to be removed. If the rectum can be preserved, the ostomy will probably be temporary, done to allow the surgical site to heal properly. After healing is complete, bowel function is restored through "reversal" surgery. The difference between temporary and permanent ostomies is explained in chapter 2.

Familial Adenomatous Polyposis (FAP)

Some people who suffer from colorectal cancer develop it because they have a hereditary disease called familial adenomatous polyposis (FAP).

The "familial" part of the name means that it runs in the family – it's genetically transmitted from generation to generation. In 1946, Dr. Eldon J. Gardner studied a Utah family in which nine members had died of colon cancer over three generations. He found that a single autosomal dominant gene was responsible. However, one-third of patients with FAP have no family history of FAP, which means that they acquired a spontaneous genetic defect instead of inheriteing the defect from their parents.

Not all children of a parent with the gene will develop the disease, but if one parent has the gene, then each of the children has a 50 percent chance of inheriting it. And children who do inherit the gene will develop colorectal cancer in adulthood – if FAP is left untreated.

What are the symptoms of FAP? Well, the disease typically begins in adolescence, at about ages ten through twelve, but it may not be diagnosed until the teens or even early twenties. Polyps (abnormal lumps of cells) begin to form in the colon or rectum. These polyps eventually develop into cancers, Most often the polyps cauuse no symptoms, or they can manifest through blood or mucus in your stool, diarrhea, occasional abdominal cramps or unexplained weight loss.

People without FAP can also develop polyps. In fact, they're rather common in people over fifty. These polyps can be pre-malignant or not, and only examination under a microscope can determine that. In contrast, people with FAP always have pre-malignant polyps.

The good news is that FAP is a precancerous, not a cancerous, condition. If it's diagnosed and treated early on, colon cancer is not inevitable. In fact, it's estimated that FAP is responsible for only one percent of all colon cancers.

Treating FAP

FAP can be treated in a number of ways, depending on the number and location of the polyps in the colon and rectum.

If there are few or no polyps in the rectum, it may be possible to remove the colon and leave the rectum. This surgery is called ileorectal anastomosis, which means that it joins the ileum with the rectum. If you get this surgery, you won't have a stoma and you won't need to wear an appliance, although your bowel movements may be much looser than before. Another option is to remove the rectum, leave the anus, and connect a small bowel pouch to the anus. Again, an external appliance will not be necessary.

Inflammatory Bowel Disease

It's estimated that about four million people worldwide (including one million Americans, 23,000 Australians and 250,000 Canadians) suffer from IBD.

The term inflammatory bowel disease (IBD) refers to both Crohn's disease and ulcerative colitis. Both are chronic intestinal disorders, which cause abdominal pain, cramping, fatigue and diarrhea.

What's the difference between Crohn's disease and ulcerative colitis? Crohn's disease causes inflammation of the lining and wall of any part of the digestive system – from the mouth to the anus. The small intestine or colon, and sometimes both, may be affected. Ulcerative colitis causes inflammation of the lining of the rectum (proctitis) and the colon (colitis).

In the case of both Crohn's disease and colitis, the lining of the intestinal wall is red and swollen, becomes ulcerated, and bleeds. However, Crohn's disease affects all three layers of the intestine, while colitis affects only the inner layers of the colon (called the mucosa and the submucosa).

Who gets IBD?

IBD can strike anyone at any time, with little preference for age, gender or race. However, people are most frequently diagnosed with IBD between the ages of 15 to 25, or 45 to 80, and IBD seems to be more common in North America and Northern Europe. There's also evidence that IBD runs in families, since approximately 15 to 30 percent of IBD sufferers have a relative with the disease.

Diet and IBD

There is some evidence linking IBD to Vitamin D deficiency, since Vitamin D deficiency is more common in people who have inflammatory bowel disease. But this may not be due entirely to diet.

The fact that IBD is more prevalent in North America and Northern Europe – regions that receive less sunlight – suggests that climate may play a role. Since Vitamin D is manufactured in the skin on exposure to sunlight, the body makes significantly less of it in northern climates, especially in winter.

The connection between smoking and IBD

Although the cause of IBD is unknown, research does show that current and former smokers have a higher risk of developing Crohn's disease than do nonsmokers. In addition, smoking is associated with a higher rate of relapse, repeat surgery and immunosuppressive treatment for people with IBD. And the risk for women is slightly higher than for men – regardless of whether the woman is a former or current smoker.

Why smoking increases the risk of Crohn's disease is unknown, but some theories suggest that smoking might lower the intestine's defenses, decrease blood flow to the area, or cause immune system changes that result in inflammation.

In contrast, colitis is less common among smokers than it is among nonsmokers and ex-smokers. Again, although the reasons for this are unknown, some research suggests that nicotine patches improve the symptoms of colitis sufferers. Unfortunately, high doses of nicotine have side efects, such as skin rashes, nausea and dizziness.

What are the symptoms of IBD?

The symptoms for Crohn's disease and colitis are similar: abdominal pain, cramping, fatigue and diarrhea. Crohn's disease may also involve a fever. Fever is usually not present for colitis sufferers unless the colon enlarges and distends. (This is a condition called toxic megacolon, and it makes immediate surgery necessary to prevent the colon from rupturing.)

Symptoms vary widely in severity, and can come and go. If you have IBD, you may experience only occasional, mild flare-ups, or you may have constant debilitating symptoms that prevent you from living a normal life. Many people experience flare-ups after periods of apparent health. If the flare-up is serious, it can result in hospitalization.

Diet, drugs and surgery are used to improve and, in some cases, eliminate symptoms, but the cause and cure of IBD is unknown. The only known cure for ulcerative colitis is surgery.

Treating IBD

Obviously, you're not going to want to consider ostomy as anything but a last resort. But if you're experiencing a severe flare-up of IBD and the inflammation doesn't respond to drug therapy, your doctor may suggest ostomy surgery.

For many people, this is anything but a welcome suggestion. But keep in mind that – when necessary – ostomy surgery will not only improve your health, but also your quality of life.

If your doctor recommends an ostomy, you're probably dealing with:

- Lots of bleeding and pain.
- A severe, long-term illness.
- An ulceration that makes a hole in the intestinal wall.
- A medical treatment plan that's not controlling the disease.
- Intestinal obstruction.

Not everyone finds the recommendation that they get ostomy surgery unwelcome. In fact, it's not uncommon for IBD sufferers who once dreaded the prospect of life with an ostomy to wonder why they waited so long to get one. If you're getting an ostomy because of IBD, don't be surprised if you experience remarkable and swift improvements in your quality of life soon after surgery.

When ostomy surgery is necessary for colitis sufferers, it often means an ileostomy that removes the diseased colon. Removal of the colon and rectum is a permanent cure, since the site of disease has been removed. You may also be a candidate for an ileorectal or ileoanal anastomosis. These surgical procedures join the ileum with either the rectum or the anus. If you get this surgery, you won't have a stoma and you won't need to wear an appliance, although your bowel movements may be much looser than before. Chapter 2 tells you more about continent procedures like ileorectal or ileoanal anastomosis.

When ostomy surgery is necessary for Crohn's disease sufferers, it's typically an ileostomy that removes the entire colon from the ileum on down, and sometimes a portion of the small intestine as well. The ileoanal anastomosis procedures aren't appropriate for treating Crohn's disease, since it's possible for the inflammation to recur in the remaining small intestine that would be used to create an internal pouch. Even a conventional ileostomy isn't a permanent cure, since the inflammation can recur elsewhere in the digestive system – anywhere from the mouth to the anus. But despite this, many Crohn's disease sufferers experience immense improvements in vitality without a recurrence of the disease.

Keep in mind, though, that you'll need to consult with your healthcare professionals – family doctor, surgeon, and Wound, Ostomy and Continence (WOC) nurse – to determine the best type of surgery for you.

2
TYPES OF OSTOMIES

What are the different types of ostomies?

Let's say your doctor has recommended that you get an ostomy. The next step is to explore this option to determine what type of ostomy surgery is right for you. There are several surgical choices, each with its own set of advantages and disadvantages.

Remember that, whatever you situation, there exist a number of options for the type of ostomy that's appropriate for you. The decision will be dictated by the extent and severity of your disease, your state of health, and whether you've had any previous resections, among other things.

Colostomy: The Basics

When you have a colostomy, the damaged or diseased portion of your colon is removed. The healthy end of the colon is brought to the surface of your abdomen, and a stoma is created. Stool is eliminated via the stoma instead of the usual route of the anus. A stoma is an artificial opening created in the surface of the body. The surface of the stoma is actually the lining of the intestine, usually appearing moist and pink. We'll look at how to care for the stoma in chapter 5. In the next few sections, we'll be talking about what colostomies, ileostomies and urostomies are. To familiarize yourself with the different parts of the digestive system, take a look at the diagram of the digestive tract on the next page.

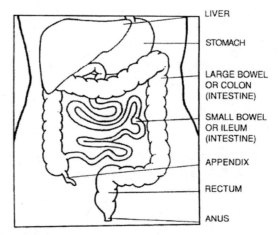

LIVER

STOMACH

LARGE BOWEL
OR COLON
(INTESTINE)

SMALL BOWEL
OR ILEUM
(INTESTINE)

APPENDIX

RECTUM

ANUS

The normal digestive tract
Copyright © United Ostomy Association of Canada Inc. Reprinted with permission.

If your doctor has recommended a colostomy, you're probably suffering from one of the following:

- cancer;
- Crohn's disease;
- diverticulitis;
- injury (or trauma to the abdominal region); or
- congenital (present at birth) conditions.

Some of these conditions can lead to an ileostomy rather than a colostomy. How is an ileostomy different from a colostomy?

In a colostomy, only part of the colon (large intestine) is surgically removed or bypassed. A stoma is created from the end of the colon that is brought through the abdomen. By contrast, in an ileostomy, the entire colon is removed or bypassed and a stoma is created from the end of the ileum. Types of ileostomies are described in the next section.

There are a number of alternative options for both colostomy and ileostomy surgery, and we'll look at these later in this chapter.

How are colostomies and ileostomies different from urostomies? A urostomy, or urinary diversion, involves the creation of a stoma that diverts urine flow from a diseased, defective or injured urinary tract. It doesn't change the function of the digestive system at all. For more about urostomies, see page 37.

Types of Colostomies

Colostomy stool can range in consistency from soft to firm, and can be passed fairly continuously or at intervals. The frequency and consistency varies depending on the person and the location of the stoma. It also varies depending on how the colostomy is managed. For example, you may choose to irrigate your colostomy to empty it at predictable and less frequent intervals. Or you may choose to wear an appliance (also called a pouch). This requires a smaller time commitment, but means that your colostomy will produce stool at less predictable intervals. It depends on what's right for you. (We'll look at the different methods of managing colostomies in chapter 5.)

Ascending colostomy

An ascending colostomy is located on the right side of the abdomen within the ascending colon. This type of colostomy is relatively rare.

Transverse colostomy

A transverse colostomy is created from the transverse portion of the colon. The stoma is located in the upper abdomen, within the transverse colon (and is usually in the central upper abdomen). This is the site of most temporary colostomies.

The stool consistency of transverse colostomies is liquid to semi-formed. It may be paste-like in consistency, because the ascending colon will have absorbed some of the fluid from the waste.

Loop and double-barrel colostomy

Most loop and double-barrel ostomies are located in the transverse colon, and are therefore a variation on the transverse colostomy. Stool consistency will vary according to where in the gastrointestinal tract the loop or double-barrel colostomy is formed. Most often, it will be liquid to semi-formed, similar to the transverse colostomy.

- A *double barrel colostomy* is created when the transverse colon is completely severed, and two separate stomas are created on the upper abdomen. The proximal stoma (the one nearest to the upper gastrointestinal tract) is the functional end that is connected to the upper gastrointestinal tract and will drain stool. The distal stoma (the one closest to the end of the gastrointestinal tract) is connected to the rectum. It is also called a mucous fistula, because it drains small amounts of mucus material. Here's a diagram of a transverse double barrel colostomy.

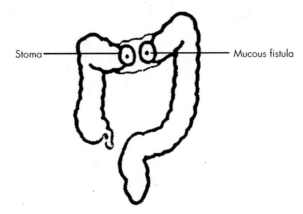

Stoma — Mucous fistula

Double barrel colostomy
Copyright © United Ostomy Association of Canada Inc. Reprinted with permission.

Both stomas can be brought out at the same spot that forms the double barrel colostomy, or separately (they're then called colostomy and mucous fistula).

- A *loop colostomy* is created by bringing a loop of bowel through an incision in the upper abdominal wall. The loop is held in place outside the abdomen by a plastic rod slipped beneath it. An incision is made in the bowel to allow the passage of stool through the loop colostomy. The supporting rod is removed approximately seven to ten days after surgery, when healing has occurred to the extent that it will prevent the loop of bowel from retracting into the abdomen. A loop colostomy is most often performed in order to create a temporary stoma to divert stool away from an area of intestine that has been blocked or ruptured. Here's a diagram of a transverse loop colostomy.

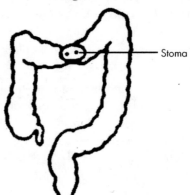

Stoma

Loop colostomy
Copyright © United Ostomy Association of Canada Inc. Reprinted with permission.

Descending colostomy

A descending colostomy is located in the descending colon. The stool consistency from a descending colostomy is fairly firm, since much of the water has been absorbed as the stool moves through the ascending and transverse colons. The stool is much less irritating to the peristomal skin than that of colostomies created further up in the gastrointestinal tract.

Sigmoid colostomy

A sigmoid colostomy is a type of descending colostomy that's created from the sigmoid portion of the colon. The functioning end of the colon (the section of bowel that remains connected to the upper gastrointestinal tract) is brought out onto the surface of the abdomen. The distal portion of bowel (the portion that's now connected only to the rectum) may be removed, or sutured closed and left in the abdomen, depending on whether it is diseased or not.

In a sigmoid colostomy, the stool is fully formed because most of the water has been absorbed as the waste passes through the remaining large bowel.

The most common types of colostomy surgery performed are the descending and sigmoid colostomies. These colostomies are often permanent, and result from trauma, cancer or other disease. Here's a diagram of a sigmoid colostomy.

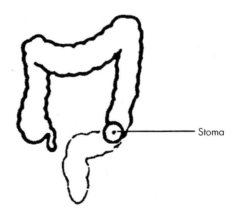

Stoma

Sigmoid colostomy
Copyright © United Ostomy Association of Canada Inc. Reprinted with permission.

Colostomy Options

A colostomy - for now or forever?

Colostomies may be either permanent or temporary. If a colostomy is temporary, the rectum, anus and at least some of the colon must be disease-free, and the surgeon must leave them intact. The temporary colostomy is created to allow the healthy parts of the bowel to heal. After healing is complete, the temporary colostomy is closed during a second operation.

For example, if you have colorectal cancer but the cancer hasn't affected your anus, it's possible that the surgeon can remove the diseased part of the colon and reconnect the healthy ends. You'll need an ostomy because stool still needs to exit the body while the reconnected parts of the colon heal. But because your anus is intact, the ostomy will be temporary.

Injury can also result in a temporary ostomy. For example, if an automobile accident results in injury to the colon, a surgeon will create a temporary ostomy to allow stool to exit the body. This temporary ostomy bypasses the injured part of the colon, giving it time to heal.

In both examples, later surgery will reconnect the healthy portions of the colon, and stool will be eliminated via the anus as before. This later surgery is called a colostomy reversal or colostomy closure.

Ileostomy: The Basics

Like colostomies, ileostomies may be temporary or permanent. But because they're created from the end of the ileum, the ileostomy stoma is usually smaller than that of a colostomy, and it's usually located on the right side of the abdomen. Also, because the ostomy is higher up in the gastrointestinal tract, the stool produced by an ileostomy is more caustic, liquid and frequent than that of a colostomy. To protect the skin from the caustic stool, the stoma usually protrudes farther from the abdominal wall that the colostomy stoma does.

If your doctor has recommended an ileostomy, you're probably suffering from one of the following conditions:

- inflammatory bowel diseases (ulcerative colitis and Crohn's disease);
- familial adenomatous polyposis (FAP);
- cancer;
- injury (or trauma to the abdominal region); or
- congenital (present at birth) conditions.

Some of these conditions can also result in a colostomy, depending on the nature and extent of the problem. Generally, an ileostomy is more common for people suffering from inflammatory bowel diseases like Crohn's disease. That's because Crohn's disease can affect the entire gastrointestinal tract, not just the colon.

Types of Ileostomies

The Brooke ileostomy is the standard, conventional type of ileostomy.

Created by surgeon Dr. Bryan Brooke (and therefore called the "Brooke ileostomy") this type of ileostomy involves removing or bypassing the entire colon, and in some cases a portion of the small intestine (e.g., in the case of Crohn's disease). The ileum is then brought to the surface of the abdomen, and a stoma is created. The stoma is usually smaller than that of a colostomy, since it's created from the small intestine rather than the colon.

The greater the length of small intestine removed, the greater the loss of nutrient absorption. This can result in nutritional deficiencies that may require adjustments to your diet. Since the colon has also been removed, you may be at risk for developing fluid and electrolyte imbalances. To prevent this, ensure that you drink plenty of fluids, especially during hot weather and sporting activities. Over time, the remaining ileum will adapt and take over part of the absorptive capabilities of the colon. See the section on dietary guidelines and nutrition on page 80 for more information. Here's a diagram of a standard (Brooke) ileostomy.

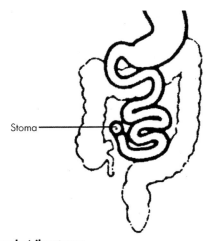

Standard (Brooke) ileostomy
Copyright © United Ostomy Association of Canada Inc. Reprinted with permission.

Ileostomy Options: The Continent Ileostomy

When ostomy surgery becomes necessary for IBD sufferers, many have experienced years of pain, bleeding, and incontinence. For those people, ostomy surgery is a saving grace — especially if the surgery will allow them to be continent without the need to wear an ostomy pouch. The continent ileostomy lets them do just that.

There are two basic types of continent ileostomies. Although neither requires the use of an external pouch, there are key differences in how each is managed.

The ileoanal reservoir (pouch) procedure

The ileoanal reservoir is not an ileostomy per se. It was developed in the last 20 years, and has become an attractive alternative to the conventional ileostomy among patients with ulcerative colitis and FAP. To construct the reservoir, the small bowel is used. Because the bowel used to make the pouch would always be at risk of developing the disease among patients with Crohn's disease, the procedure isn't performed in these patients (except in very rare circumstances). The pouch is most often "J" shaped, but it can be "W" or "S" shaped as well. The latter shapes are slightly roomier, but their function is the same. Here's a diagram of an ileoanal reservoir (pelvic pouch).

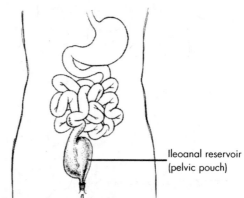

Ileoanal reservoir
(pelvic pouch)

Ileoanal reservoir (pelvic pouch)
Copyright © United Ostomy Association of Canada Inc. Reprinted with permission.

Whatever its shape, the pouch provides a storage place for stool, since the colon is no longer available for the job. Since the anal sphincter muscles are still intact, they hold in the stool until you're ready to pass it. About four to six times per day and one or two times per night, you'll pass stool through the anus. Keep in mind that stool frequency will increase in the first few weeks following surgery, but it settles down after that and remains stable. Although there are no specific dietary restrictions with an ileoanal reservoir, you may decide to avoid certain foods known to increase stool frequency, such as caffeine. See the section on dietary guidelines and nutrition on page 80 for more information.

Ileoanal reservoir surgery is a favorite because it eliminates both the disease and the need for a permanent ileostomy. Surgery may be performed in one, two or three stages; however, it's most often done in two. Each stage is typically two to three months apart. The first stage removes the colon (but leaves the anus intact); constructs a pouch from a portion of the small intestine; and creates a temporary ileostomy. The temporary ileostomy lets the surgical incisions heal. Two to three months later, the bowel is reconnected to the now-healed pouch, and the temporary ileostomy is closed.

Jon, 29, has this to say about the ileoanal reservoir procedure:

After being diagnosed with ulcerative colitis four years ago, I began taking prednisone and many other drugs to control the symptoms. My symptoms were severe and drugs didn't really work. They'd work for a while (and I'd suffer from their side effects) but then I'd get sick from the colitis again. I was using the toilet 20 to 30 times per day, and I had no control over it. It was truly awful. I eventually had to go on a disability leave from my job as a software developer. I really didn't want to get an ostomy, but when my doctor told me about J-pouch surgery, I decided to give it a try. I had two operations. During the first one, my colon was removed and a J-pouch was created. I also got a temporary ileostomy. About five weeks after the surgery, I went for an x-ray, which showed that my J-pouch had healed up. The surgeon said that this meant they could do the second and final operation. During that operation, my ileostomy was closed and the J-pouch was connected. I'm doing great now, thanks! Even though I still need to use the toilet five/ six times per day, as well as twice at night, I'm now able to control it. With colitis, I had no control at all.

Like Jon's, your quality of life stands a good chance of improving with this procedure.

This procedure is also called a J-pouch, pullthrough, endorectal pullthrough, pelvic pouch, or some combination of these terms.

Continent intestinal reservoir (Koch pouch)

In 1969, Swedish surgeon Nils Koch introduced another type of continent ileostomy: the Koch pouch or continent intestinal reservoir. As illustrated in the following patients, the Koch pouch is a very attractive idea for patients who no longer have an anus. However, it should be noted that because of the complexity of the procedure and the frequent complications, this pouch is constructed by only a few surgeons, and only in specialized centers.

In this type of continent ileostomy, the surgeon creates a reservoir inside the abdomen from a portion of the ileum. A narrow stoma then extends from the reservoir to the abdomen. The stoma is small, and flush with the skin. It doesn't protrude from the skin as it does with a conventional ileostomy. The reservoir is "self-sealing" – that is, it stores waste internally, and is continent. Continence is sustained by the presence of a one-way valve that keeps stool from coming out. The reservoir usually has the capacity to hold 500 – 1000 ml of stool. People with this type of ileostomy insert a catheter two to four times per day to drain the reservoir. The reservoir can be emptied anywhere, including public bathrooms. Many people choose to cover the stoma with a small pad of adhesive dressing, since mucus accumulates at the opening. Here's a diagram of a continent intestinal reservoir.

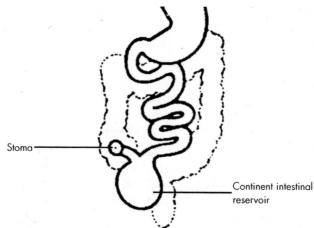

Continent intestinal reservoir
Copyright © United Ostomy Association of Canada Inc. Reprinted with permission.

Continent intestinal reservoir surgery can improve absorption, eliminate skin irritation, and prevent ileostomy problems associated with conventional ileostomies such as hernia and prolapse. It also has the lifestyle advantages of eliminating the external pouch, as well as unexpected leaks, noise and gas.

Who gets this type of ileostomy? People with conventional Brooke ileostomies sometimes choose to convert to this type of ileostomy for medical and lifestyle reasons. (It tends to alleviate, for example, severe skin problems around the stoma.) Or, people who can't have an ileoanal reservoir because their rectum and anus must be removed may elect to have intestinal reservoir surgery instead.

And some people who've had the ileoanal reservoir procedure discussed above have unacceptable diarrhea and incontinence and require an ileostomy for control. For these people, continent intestinal reservoir may be a better surgical option.

This was the case for Michele, 31:

> I converted from my J-pouch to a Koch pouch because I was going to the bathroom 10 to15 times per day with my J-pouch, which I really hated because it kept me from doing pretty much everything. It's definitely difficult to adjust to the catheter. But now I can go three to four hours without using the bathroom and for me, that's an enormous improvement.

The continent ileostomy doesn't work for everyone, though. Although continent intestinal reservoir surgery is often appropriate for individuals with colitis, it's usually not an option for those with Crohn's disease. The reason is that Crohn's disease tends to recur in the reservoir, which must then be removed. If too much of the small intestine is removed, the Crohn's disease sufferer runs the risk of developing short bowel syndrome, in which there isn't enough small intestine left to absorb sufficient nutrients.

A continent ileostomy is also not an option if you are:

- Elderly or severely overweight.
- Suffer from malnutrition or experience severe side effects with steroid therapy. Keep in mind, though, that a standard ileostomy may be converted to an ileoanal anastomosis once the body grows stronger if the rectum is left intact.

Possible problems with continent ileostomies

Although most people are happy with their continent ileostomies, there are some potential problems as well.

With intestinal reservoir surgery, sometimes the one-way valve fails to work properly, making the ileostomy incontinent or difficult to empty.

However, this problem is increasingly uncommon due to improvements in surgical technique.

- Pouchitis, or inflammation of the lining of the pouch, may also be a problem with continent ileostomy surgery. It can be a long term problem for some, but most cases can be cleared up with antibiotics.
- With pelvic pouch surgery, pouchitis symptoms include a steadily increasing stool frequency (up to eight or more per day), bleeding, abdominal cramping, fever, and an urgent need to defecate.
- If you have a Koch pouch, you may also find that the ileostomy stool is more watery (making it necessary that you intubate the pouch more frequently), and occasionally, there may be blood in the stool.
- Other side effects or complications may include small intestinal obstruction with abdominal bloating, incontinence or leaking.

These complications are treatable if dealt with promptly, and hospital staff is trained to observe and handle them. However, frequent episodes of pouchitis and other complications of continent ileostomies may have to be resolved by removing the pouch and creating a conventional end ileostomy. But if you have a pelvic pouch and are experiencing problems linked specifically to the pouch, keep in mind that you may be able to convert to a continent reservoir ileostomy (meaning that you may not have to resort to a conventional ileostomy). Always discuss your options with your doctor.

An Ileostomy – For Now or Forever?

For some people, ileostomies are temporary. For example, if you're getting one of the alternative options, such as the ileoanal reservoir procedure, you'll have a temporary ostomy with an external stoma, so you'll need to know how to care for it. Ileoanal reservoir surgery is described on page 32.

Another reason why it's a good idea to learn to deal with your ostomy is that it's possible your surgeon may not be able to create an ileoanal reservoir during the latter part of the ileoanal reservoir surgery. This is what happened to Tom:

> My ileostomy wasn't supposed to be permanent. I was supposed to get a J-pouch, but after the surgeon saw my colon during surgery, he said there was too much damage from my colitis that he couldn't give me the J-pouch. Well, I've just celebrated my first anniversary with my permanent ostomy. Would I do it again if I knew the outcome? Definitely! Now I can go places where there

might not even be a bathroom, and I never have to worry about eating the foods that used to give me flare-ups. But I'm not going to kid you – some days, it just doesn't feel great to have an ostomy. There are good days, and there are bad days. But I will tell you that once you get over that recovery time and find an appliance that works for you, you can live each day knowing you won't be in pain.

Urostomy: The Basics

Although all three types of ostomies involve the creation of an external stoma on the abdomen, in the case of a urostomy, or urinary diversion, the stoma diverts urine flow from a diseased, defective or injured urinary tract. It does not affect the passage of stool from the digestive system.

If your doctor has suggested a urostomy, you're probably suffering from one of the following conditions:

- cancer (probably the most common reason);
- injury (or trauma to the abdominal region);
- congenital (present at birth) conditions;
- infections;or
- other blockages that can't be managed by less invasive measures.

Types of Urostomies

Ileal conduit

The most common type of urostomy is the ileal conduit. It's also called the ileal loop or Bricker's loop, after the surgeon who developed the procedure.

To create the ileal conduit, a surgeon will separate a small section of the ileum from the rest of the small intestine to create a short tube. One end of the tube is sewn shut and the other end is brought to the surface of the abdomen. To allow the urine to flow through this tube, the ureters are attached to the tube. Urine now flows outside the body into an external pouch. The pouch is emptied several times per day.

To complete the surgery, the two ends of the small intestine are reconnected to allow stool to pass as it did before. So, although the urostomy is formed from a small section of the ileum, it doesn't change the function of the digestive system. Here's a diagram of a standard urostomy (ileal conduit).

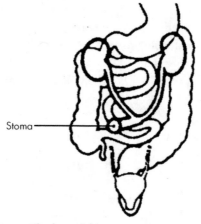

Standard urostomy (ileal conduit)
Copyright © United Ostomy Association of Canada Inc. Reprinted with permission.

Colonic conduit

Sometimes a portion of the colon is used instead of the ileum to create the conduit. This is called a colonic conduit. It's also called a cecal conduit, since it's usually the first part of the colon, or cecum, that is used to create the conduit. It functions in the same way as the ileal conduit — it's simply a passageway for urine. Again, to complete the surgery, the two ends of the colon are reconnected and the function of the digestive system remains unchanged.

The ileal and colonic conduits are simply passageways for the urine, and no more. Although they work well for many people, there are several problems associated with them.

For example, urine may "back up" into the kidneys and cause infection. That's why people with urostomies must be very careful in maintaining their ostomies to stop this from happening. Also, unlike other types of ostomies involving the digestive tract, urostomies are almost never inactive. Normally, the kidneys produce several drops of urine every minute, so urine is always flowing. Proper care is needed to avoid leakage and keep urine from flowing backward into the conduit, and possibly infecting the kidneys.

The good news is that with proper care and attention, these problems are unlikely to occur. We'll look at how to care for your urostomy in the next chapter.

Urostomy Options

Although the standard surgery for urostomies is still the ileal conduit, there are alternatives. The most common of these is the internal continent reservoir, or continent urostomy. Several variations exist. Each involves the creation of a reservoir inside the abdomen. The reservoir is created with either a portion of small intestine or the colon. The pouch has a one-way valve inside it that holds in the urine. To drain the pouch, a catheter is inserted four to six times per day. Examples of internal continent reservoirs are the Koch, Indiana, Mainz, Miami, Studer, and Mitrofanoff pouches. Here's a diagram of an internal continent reservoir (continent urostomy).

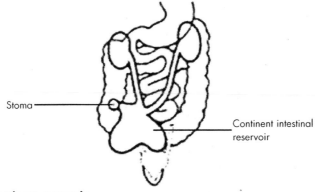

Internal continent reservoir
Copyright © United Ostomy Association of Canada Inc. Reprinted with permission.

Less common alternatives to a standard urostomy include a substitute bladder (also called an orthotopic bladder or neobladder) and the rectal reservoir.

A substitute bladder is an internal reservoir created from a portion of the small intestine. It connects directly to the urethra, so that urine flows out of the body via the urethra. Another name for this is the ileal neobladder, since the pouch is made from the small intestine (ileum). Because there is no stoma, there is no need for an external appliance – urine is voided naturally through the urethra, though it may take several months to achieve continence. This can mean greater satisfaction and fewer changes to your body image. In fact, studies suggest that patients with substitute bladders experience better psychosocial adjustment than patients with diversions requiring external collection devices.

Remember, though, that not everyone is a candidate for this type of surgery. Because neobladder surgery can take between four and eight hours (depending on the type of procedure used), you really need to be in good health overall to undergo the procedure. You also need to have the motor control and dexterity required to perform self-catheterization, if necessary, and have the patience and determination to learn how to empty your new bladder.

In the rectal reservoir option, a small pouch is constructed and connected to the rectum. Urine exits the body via the rectum, along with stool. Valves in the reservoir protect the kidneys from the bacteria that can exist in urine backflow, and in the rectum.

As with other types of ostomy surgery, you'll need to consult with your healthcare professionals – family doctor, surgeon, and WOC nurse – to determine the best procedure for you.

Possible problems with continent urostomies

Continent reservoirs are more complex procedures than the ileal or colonic conduits, which means that they require a longer recovery time and intensive postoperative care. They are also more prone to complications.

Possible problems include pouchitis (probably the most common), scarring, obstruction of the ureters, chronic urinary tract infections and problems with self-catheterization. The good news is that with proper care, all of these potential problems are readily treatable.

A Urostomy – For Now or Forever?

Like colostomies and ileostomies, a urostomy may be temporary, carried out to allow diseased or injured tissue a chance to heal. For example, a temporary urostomy may be created for a child born with a defect of the urinary tract. Ostomy surgery is performed immediately after birth, and corrective surgery is then done at a later date, when the child's body is big enough to handle it. For many children, this may mean that most of the childhood years are spent with an ostomy; for others, the corrective surgery can be done more quickly. See "Babies and Children With Ostomies" on page 129 for more information.

3
BEFORE OSTOMY SURGERY

When you're preparing for ostomy surgery, there's a lot to think about. The one thing you'll almost certainly have in common with anyone who has ever prepared for ostomy surgery is apprehension. If you're feeling anxious and fearful, then take heart. Your apprehension is natural and normal – anyone in your shoes would be experiencing the same emotions. But while ostomy surgery is undeniably life-changing, the 21st century is a very good time for you to be going through it. Surgical techniques, as well as pre- and post-operative care, have improved to the point where ostomy operations are routinely successful.

This chapter's goal is to provide information that will allay your pre-surgery fears and give you techniques to handle your recovery. While pre-operative care is similar for all types of ostomies, post-operative care and rehabilitation vary, depending on whether you're getting a conventional ostomy or one of the continent procedures.

The most important thing to remember for both before and after ostomy surgery is that it's your body. This means that you're ultimately in control of it and responsible for it. Although there will doubtless be times during the pre-and post-surgical periods when you feel that your body is out of your control, it's important to realize that you deserve all the information you need to understand what's happening to you and why. Taking charge of what's happening to you will make you feel less apprehensive and more confident, ensuring your successful recovery from ostomy surgery.

That's not to say that it won't take time for you to adjust to your ostomy. It's totally normal and acceptable for you to ask *"why me?"* and to explore answers to that question. But at the same time, it will benefit you to cultivate a "take charge" attitude wherever possible. Attitude alone can't cure chronic IBD or colorectal cancer – in some cases, ostomy surgery is the only thing that will help. But believing that you're in control of your body *and* your life will both help reduce your fear of the surgery and support you in your recovery process.

Robin, 55, who had surgery for colorectal cancer, says the following:

> I was definitely scared of the surgery and what might happen. I was scared of the surgery itself. I was scared of the pain I would feel when I woke up. I was scared of waking up with an ugly stoma with a pouch attached to it. And I was even scared of never waking up at all! But my healthcare team was great. My surgeon explained to me what was going to happen during surgery, and told me that I would be getting painkillers to deal with any pain I felt. My WOC nurse and I discussed what my stoma would look like after surgery and how I would learn to take care of it. They both assured me that ostomy surgery is routine and successful surgery, and I had the best possible chances of a smooth recovery. As it turns out, they were right. Here I am, a year later, and I'm doing great. I think the most important thing you can do before any type of surgery is get the answers to all your questions. Don't be afraid to ask!

To help you develop a take charge attitude, read the "Ostomate's Bill of Rights" reprinted at the end of this chapter.

Preparing for Ostomy Surgery

Well before your surgery, you should meet with your team of healthcare providers to get an understanding of what to expect. The only time when this may not be possible is if your surgery is an emergency. In that case, all the explanations as to what happens during surgery and why will come after the surgery has been completed, when you're recovering.

Generally, your healthcare team will include you (of course!) as well as a number of specialists: your family doctor; your gastroenterologist or urologist; a Wound, Ostomy and Continence (WOC) nurse; and the surgeon who'll be performing the surgery. A gastroenterologist is a medical doctor who specializes in treating diseases of the gastrointestinal (digestive) tract, and a urologist is a medical doctor who specializes in treating diseases of the urinary tract. A WOC is a registered nurse who specializes in ostomy care. He or she is specially trained to instruct on correct care of the ostomy, suggest suitable appliances, and help with the psychological and emotional adjustment to life with an ostomy. You may also see a WOC referred to as an ET, or Enterostomal Therapist. These are different names for the same thing.

Despite the fact that you're obviously the most important member of your healthcare team, throughout this chapter, I'll be using the term "healthcare team" to refer mainly to your WOC nurse, gastroenterologist or urologist, and surgeon.

In addition to your healthcare team, you may also benefit from talking to someone who's already gone through the type of ostomy surgery you'll be having. It can be very encouraging to talk to someone who's not only survived but also *thrived* from getting an ostomy. The United Ostomy Association offers a service that arranges visits from those who best match your situation. Check the Resources section of this book for contact information.

Your healthcare team – or a member of it – will likely provide you with written information (such as booklets and pamphlets). Written information can go a long way toward relieving your fears about the surgery, because it explains what to expect both before and after surgery. It's often difficult to retain all of the information given to you orally, and written information can be referred to again and again. Your relatives and close friends may also want to read the information, if they're going to be involved in your recovery and rehabilitation. Many excellent brochures, booklets, care manuals, and videos are available from the United Ostomy Association. For more information, contact your local UOA chapter, or go to the website at *www.uoa.org/*.

If someone close to you will be caring for your ostomy along with (or instead of) you, it's crucial that they be involved in all educational activities.

You should also take the opportunity to ask any questions that you may have about the surgery and recovery. Your healthcare team has a responsibility to respond to your questions. The more organized you are and the more clear about your concerns and questions, the better able they will be to respond to them. So that's why it's a good idea to write down both your questions and the answers provided by your healthcare team. You may even want to tape their answers, if you aren't good at taking notes and talking to people at the same time. The more specific you can be about what you want to know, the better your chances will be of getting the answers you need.

Preparation Q&A

Here are some questions and issues you should address with your healthcare team before your surgery.

Can you provide me with information about what to expect from my surgery?

Hospitals generally provide information about ostomy surgery and ostomy care in several forms. Ask your WOC nurse, doctor or surgeon for patient guides, pamphlets, videos and any other information they may have available.

Some hospitals provide a general guide to preparing for surgery that gives patients and their families an overview about what will happen before, during, and after surgery. They also offer additional patient guides explaining what happens in the different types of ostomy surgery. These patient guides also include dietary guidelines, basic ostomy care instructions, and information about where to buy ostomy supplies. Taken together, these resources provide the hospital's patients with a good idea of what to expect. Ask if your hospital offers something similar.

But written material isn't enough. Well before your surgery, you should see a video about caring for a stoma. If a video isn't available, a diagram also works well, if combined with an explanation from your WOC nurse. A model stoma is an even better tool to help the WOC nurse teach you how to how to apply and empty the pouch, clean the stoma, and take care of the skin around the stoma. Ask if your hospital makes these types of educational tools available.

This is critical even if you're getting a continent ileostomy, since you'll need to care for your temporary ileostomy yourself between stages (that is, between the ileostomy formation and the "takedown" procedure).

Many people find that it's often difficult to absorb this education before and directly after surgery. Some are too preoccupied by fears and anxieties to absorb much before the surgery, and too exhausted and medicated to absorb it directly afterward. Request that these instructions for managing an ostomy be repeated when you're further into your recovery process, and even after you've returned home.

If a close relative or friend will be helping you recover from surgery and/or care for the ostomy, it's a good idea for them to be involved in this education, too. That means that they should be involved in any meetings you have with your healthcare team, and they should be around to review any available videotapes or written material as well. If that person will actually be caring for your ostomy (i.e., changing pouches, etc.) then he or she should also be involved in any educational sessions you have with your WOC nurse.

It's also useful to explore other sources for written information and videos. For example, many excellent brochures, booklets, care manuals and videos are available from the United Ostomy Association. For more information, contact your local UOA chapter, or visit their website at *www.uoa.org/*.

What type of ostomy will I be getting?

This question is fundamental and should be addressed clearly by your healthcare team.

You should, of course, be informed about whether you're having an ileostomy, colostomy, or urostomy (refer back to chapter 1 if you're not sure about these terms). The answer to the question "What type of ostomy should I be getting?" should also include a clear indication of:

- whether the ostomy will be temporary or permanent;
- whether the rectum will be left intact or not; and
- whether a continent procedure, such as a J-pouch, is a possibility for you.

Sometimes, it may be difficult for your healthcare team to tell you with 100 percent certainty that your ostomy will be temporary. For example, a surgeon may attempt to remove diseased parts of the colon, then rejoin the disease-free portions. But once the surgery is underway, that surgeon may find that there isn't enough healthy tissue left to do this. At that point, a permanent ostomy will be necessary.

Even if you're scheduled for a temporary ostomy, make sure you understand the likelihood of having a permanent ostomy by discussing the chances with your WOC nurse and surgeon.

What about the location of my stoma?

Your WOC nurse or surgeon, or both, should meet with you before your surgery to determine the best placement for your stoma.

Stoma location depends to some extent on the type of ostomy you're getting. Ask your WOC nurse and surgeon what the possible locations for your stoma are based on what type of ostomy you'll be getting. For example, if you have a colostomy on the ascending colon, the stoma is located on the lower right side of the abdomen; if you have a colostomy on the descending colon, the stoma is located on the lower left side. Loop and double-barrel ostomies are variations on the transverse colostomy, so they're often located on the upper abdomen.

Because ileostomies are created from a portion of the ileum or small intestine, they're generally located on the lower right side of the abdomen. This protects the stoma when the knee is flexed, making the pouch less conspicuous.

As for urostomies, ileal or colonic conduits are typically located on the abdomen in the right-lower quadrant just below your waist and to the right of your navel.

Although stoma location is determined to some extent by the type of ostomy you're getting, your healthcare team should also do the following:

- observe your body while you're standing, sitting, twisting and lying down to determine the best place on the abdominal wall to locate the stoma; and
- mark one or more sites on your abdomen, so that the surgeon knows where to place the stoma during surgery.

Generally, the stoma should:

- be located away from scars, creases, and bony parts of the abdomen, such as ribs and hips;
- be easy for you to see, so that caring for your stoma is made easier;
- be kept within the rectus muscle, if possible, to prevent peristomal hernias;
- be "budded" to allow proper pouch placement. In general, the stoma should be approximately 1 to 1.5 inches long so that waste doesn't get between the appliance and onto the skin (this is particularly important for ileostomies, since the stool can be very caustic); and
- not be located in the midline.

To ensure that your healthcare team addresses all issues around stoma placement, you may want to ask the following questions.

1. Does my weight affect the location of the stoma?
2. Does my occupation affect the location of the stoma?
3. Do scars, skin folds, edges of the ribcage or the margins of the rectus abdominus muscle affect the site of the stoma?
4. Does a walking disability affect the placement and care of the stoma site?
5. Does previous radiation therapy affect the location of a stoma?
6. Does a previous abdominal procedure affect the location of a stoma?

What will my stoma look like?

Stoma size and shape varies. Your stoma may be round or oval; it may stick out (a budded stoma) or be flat (a flush stoma). Size and shape often depend on the type of ostomy you're getting. Ask your WOC nurse and surgeon what you should expect in your particular situation.

The stoma is warm and moist, like the inside of your mouth. It should always be a deep red or pink color, and may bleed when washed or touched; this is normal. However, if you notice a large amount of blood, contact your doctor or your WOC nurse.

Also, because the stoma has no nerve endings, it's not painful when touched. As a result, you should protect it from sharp objects, such as seat belts, and large belt buckles.

Be aware that your stoma will change in size throughout your life with weight gains or losses. This change will be most noticeable in the first six to eight weeks after surgery. Surgery causes swelling. As the swelling decreases your stoma size will decrease. Therefore, it is important for you to measure your stoma and fit the pouch opening according to size weekly. Your WOC nurse will show you how to do this.

How will I take care of my ostomy?

Written information should be provided to you that will advise you about ostomy care. It doesn't, however, replace one-on-one instruction. Your WOC nurse should be available before and after your surgery to step you through the process of caring for your ostomy. See chapters 5, 6 and 7 for basic ostomy care instructions.

Where do I get ostomy supplies?

In the days directly following surgery, ostomy supplies will be provided for you by the hospital, and your WOC nurse will manage your ostomy for you. Again, the literature provided by your hospital or local branch of the United Ostomy Association should contain this information. If you are not sure, ask your WOC nurse.

Should I stop taking immunsuppressant drugs prior to my ostomy surgery?

If you're having ostomy surgery because of IBD, you may be taking immunsuppressant drugs such as azathioprine, 6-mercaptopurine, or cyclosporine to control your symptoms. Some doctors suggest that these drugs be discontinued for three to four weeks prior to surgery because they may interfere with the healing of the tissue. Ask your healthcare team if this is appropriate in your case.

Do I have to stop smoking before my ostomy surgery?

You probably won't have to ask this question of your healthcare team! Instead, you'll likely be informed early on that you should stop smoking for as long as you can before surgery. Generally, smokers should stop smoking five to seven days before surgery — or longer, if possible. As with other types of surgery that require general anesthesia, ostomy surgery is hard on the lungs. It irritates lung tissue, making the lungs produce excess mucus. If you smoke, your lungs are already irritated and producing more mucus than normal. The good news is that if you stop smoking even for a few days before your ostomy surgery, your lungs will have a chance to recover and your chances of experiencing lung-related complications during and after surgery will substantially decrease.

Remember – it's your body and you are responsible for it. Even if you can't imagine giving up smoking permanently (especially when you're undergoing such a stressful time in your life), you'll be doing yourself a great favor if you stop smoking at least five to seven days before your surgery.

What else can I do to prepare for surgery?

Since you're probably fairly anxious about surgery, taking care of yourself both physically and emotionally is extremely important. Talking to your healthcare team about any questions you have about surgery is undoubtedly crucial to keep you feeling in charge of what's happening to you.

There are other ways to maintain your physical and mental health prior to surgery as well. For example, some complementary therapies, such as homeopathy and aromatherapy, can support you when you're getting ready for surgery.

In general, it's best to keep your healthcare team informed about any complementary therapy you decide to explore. But because these therapies are gentle and non-invasive, it's unlikely that your healthcare team will have any objections to your trying them.

Let's look at homeopathy first, since it's most applicable to helping you deal with surgery and its aftermath.

Pre-Surgery Homeopathy and Aromatherapy

Homeopathy

Homeopathic medicines have been taken for hundreds of years to alleviate both physical and emotional difficulties before and after surgery. In fact, it's been suggested (although not scientifically proven) that homeopathic medicines may reduce complications of surgery and augment healing, allowing you to recover more quickly afterward.

Homeopathic medicine is based on the principle of similars – the notion that "like cures like." The idea is that a substance that causes symptoms in large doses can cure those same symptoms in specially prepared, exceedingly small doses. These small doses stimulate your body's healing powers. Modern vaccinations, such as the flu or allergy vaccine, are based on a similar principle: small doses of bacteria or viruses are used to stimualte the immune system to create antibodies that protect against infection

And while your healthcare team will ask you not to take any food, drink or drugs prior to surgery, there have never been any reported problems related to the taking of homeopathic remedies prior to surgery. If you're not sure, consult a homeopath or other health professional trained in homeopathy for more information.

How should you take homeopathic medicines? Here are some guidelines:

- Homeopathic medicines are available in three forms: liquid, tablet and pellet (granule) form. These are readily available from most health food stores.
- It's best not to take them with food or drink – allow about twenty minutes after your last food or drink before you take them.
- If you're taking a medicine in pellet or tablet form, avoid handling the granules to prevent contamination. Instead, tip them into the cap of the container or use a clean spoon to pop them into your mouth. Then allow the pellets or granules to dissolve in your mouth or under your tongue.
- The frequency of the dose and the potency of the medicine may vary according to the type of condition. The potency of the medicine is denoted by a number, which follows its name. For example, *Aconitum* is available in a potency of 6 or 30. Keep in mind that a higher number, or potency, doesn't necessarily mean that the medicine is better for you. In general, finding the right remedy for your condition is more important than potency.
- Keep homeopathic medicines in a cool, dark place away from strong smelling substances and they'll remain effective for several years.

According to *The Consumer's Guide to Homeopathy*, by Dana Ullman, the following two homeopathic remedies may be taken before surgery:

1. Some homeopaths recommend *Ferrum phos* (6) four times a day for two days, prior to surgery in order to prevent infection and hemorrhaging.

2. Homeopathic medicines can also help you deal with emotional difficulties prior to surgery. *Gelsemium* (6 or 30) is a common remedy for those who experience great anxiety, apprehension, weakness, and trembling prior to surgery. *Aconitum* (6 or 30) is also useful in these cases.

Keep in mind that it's imperative to discuss all homeopathic medicines with your surgeon before you decide to take them.

Aromatherapy

First, a word of caution: while many people use aromatherapy essential oils such as tea tree oil and lavender to help heal minor burns, cuts and insect bites, you should avoid applying these oils directly to your abdominal area before surgery and, after surgery, to the stoma or the incision. The stoma and the skin directly around it requires specialized care with products designed strictly for that purpose. You should also avoid taking aromatherapy oils internally.

That said, aromatherapy can help you relax and feel more comfortable during the anxious days and hours before surgery.

What is aromatherapy? Briefly, aromatherapy is a healing therapy developed from the notion that essential oils (the pure, distilled aromatic oils of certain plants) taken from aromatic plants and trees can promote the health of both body and mind. One of the nice things about aromatherapy is that, when used properly, it's effective without leading to side effects. That's because the healing oils are absorbed into your bloodstream in tiny amounts that alleviate symptoms without overpowering you.

The suggestions given here are gentle enough that you can use them without having to worry about how they may interact with any pharmaceutical drugs you're taking. Despite this, it's best that you inform your healthcare team if you decide to explore aromatherapy.

Here are some suggestions for using essential oils to relax you and relieve general anxiety, agitation and sleeplessness before surgery:

- If you're having trouble sleeping or relaxing, convince someone (perhaps a spouse or friend) to give you an aromatherapy massage before bedtime or whenever you feel anxious. On the night before surgery, it's best not to massage the abdominal area with oils– the residue may interfere with the surgeon's work. Stick to the upper body area (neck and shoulders, for example) and you'll still enjoy the healing benefits of the essential oils. A foot massage can also be extremely relaxing. But at any other time, either before or after surgery, a gentle massage of the abdominal area with soothing aromatherapy massage oil can be extremely calming for an upset digestive system. Just remember not to apply the oil directly to the stoma or the skin around it.

- For a general relaxation massage, combine 6 drops of bergamot oil, 5 drops of lavender oil, 5 drops of sandalwood oil, 2 drops of chamomile oil, and 1 drop of frankincense oil to 2 ounces of vegetable oil. Any vegetable oil, such as canola or grapeseed oil from the grocery store, will do. If you don't want to make your own massage formula, ready-made "relaxation" massage formulas are available from many drug and health food stores.

- If you can't convince anyone to give you a massage, put a couple of drops of either chamomile or lavender on your pillow or on a tissue. Lay your head down and inhale deeply – you'll soon be so relaxed, you'll be off to never-never land!

Other Considerations Before Ostomy Surgery

Besides the questions you need to ask your healthcare team, you may also want to take care of the following additional issues before going in for your ostomy surgery.

- Inform your employer of the date of your surgery. Find out if you're eligible for short-term disability leave, if you need it. Some people can cover the time required for surgery and recovery with accumulated sick leave. If you do need short-term disability leave, you'll probably need a note from your doctor explaining that you'll be having surgery. You don't need to tell them the type of surgery if you don't want to. The note should include how long you're likely to be absent from work. When you return to work, you may need a release form from your doctor, stating that you're well enough for work. Don't forget to ask for these, and remember to keep a copy for yourself.

- Discuss your ostomy surgery with your insurance company. Some insurance companies require that they be informed before you go into the hospital. Be sure to do this, since your insurance company may deny benefits if you don't inform them prior to your surgery.

- Before you go in to the hospital, make sure everything is ready at home for your return. For example:
  - Stock your freezer, refrigerator, and pantry with soft, low-fiber foods.
  - Place your furniture and other necessary items carefully, to minimize trips up and down stairs.
  - Ensure that all your bills are paid, so that you don't have to worry about them when you're recovering from surgery.

Pre-Surgery Procedures to Expect

Knowing the standard pre-surgery procedures can also ease many of your fears about ostomy surgery. Some hospitals have patient guides that tell you in detail what to expect both before and after surgery. Ask if your hospital makes this information available.

To begin with, your healthcare team will record your complete medical history. This includes any previous operations, experiences with anesthesia, current medications, and allergies to medications.

You'll also receive a complete physical examination, which will include a blood work, a chemical profile, a urinalysis, blood clotting studies, a chest x-ray, and, possibly, an electrocardiogram (ECG). Your doctor may order other tests as needed.

If you're having ostomy surgery due to long term, severe IBD, it is likely that your body hasn't been getting enough nutrients. If your physical exam indicates that you have nutritional deficiencies, your doctor may recommend an evaluation by a nutritionist. If necessary, you'll be asked to start a supplemental nutrition program, which can involve anything from the addition of a high-calorie liquid drink to total parenteral nutrition (TPN). TPN is a complete form of nutrition administered via an intravenous infusion. It helps your body get the nutrients it needs to cope with surgery.

If you've been taking long-term corticosteroids, you'll be given an intravenous or intramuscular injection before, during, and for several days after surgery. And, as mentioned previously, since immunsuppressant drugs can interfere with the healing of the wound, you may be advised to stop taking these medications.

As surgery nears, you'll progress from a low-fiber diet to a clear liquid diet. To clean your gastrointestinal tract and prepare it for surgery, you'll probably be given an enema combined with oral laxatives, or you'll be required to drink a large volume of a liquid laxative. This clears out any remnants of feces, as well as the bacteria (both friendly and unfriendly) that live in the colon. After midnight the day before your surgery, you'll be told that you should not eat or drink anything else. This is called "nothing by mouth," or NPO.

As you can see, the days leading up to your surgery will be busy. But once you've completed all the preparations, you can rest assured that you and your healthcare team have done everything possible to ensure a successful surgery and a smooth recovery.

Charter of Ostomate's Rights

First issued in 1993 by the International Ostomy Association (IOA), the following charter outlines succinctly the support you can expect as a person with an ostomy.

It's the declared objective of the International Ostomy Association that all ostomates "shall have the right to a satisfactory quality of life after their surgery and that this charter shall be realized in all countries of the world."

Ostomates shall:

1. Receive pre-operative counseling to ensure that they are fully aware of the benefits of the operation and the essential facts about living with a stoma.

2. Have a well-constructed stoma placed at an appropriate site, and with full and proper consideration to the comfort of the patient.

3. Receive experienced and professional medical support and stoma nursing care in the preoperative and postoperative period both in hospital and in their community.

4. Receive full and impartial information about all relevant supplies and products available in their country.

5. Have the opportunity to choose from the available variety of ostomy management products without prejudice or constraint.

6. Be given information about their National Ostomy Association and the services and support that can be provided.

7. Receive support and information for the benefit of the family, personal caregivers and friends to increase their understanding of the

conditions and adjustments, which are necessary for achieving a satisfactory standard of life with a stoma.

8. Receive assurance that personal information regarding ostomy surgery will be treated with discretion and confidentiality to maintain privacy.

4

AFTER OSTOMY SURGERY

In Hospital and After

D irectly after your ostomy surgery, you'll probably be sleeping off the general anesthesia. However, you can expect nurses to wake you frequently with requests to breathe in deeply and cough. Although this may be annoying, it does have a purpose: to clear your lungs of excess mucus that has gathered there as a result of the anesthesia. General anesthetic is hard on your lungs: it irritates them, inducing them to produce excess mucus in response. Expelling this mucus is crucial, and to do this, you must cough. Breathing deeply and coughing will likely be uncomfortable for you, due to the incisions in your abdomen.

Usually the most comfortable position for this activity is to lie back with the head of the bed raised. You may also want to try holding a pillow over your abdominal incisions to support them while you cough.

To further help you recover from the general anesthesia, you may be given oxygen. Oxygen also helps heal your wound.

Before long (usually the day after surgery) you'll also be asked to get up and walk. This helps your circulation and breathing. The exercise also encourages the bowels to start working again.

You'll also have an IV (intravenous) tube attached to a vein in your hand or arm. The IV provided you with fluid and medications during the operation, and you'll need it to continue to do this until your digestive system starts working again.

You may also have a tube that goes through your nose and down into your stomach. This is a nasogastric (NG) tube, and it removes gas and digestive secretions that aren't needed since your body isn't digesting anything at the moment. Instead of a NG tube, you may have a gastrostomy tube, which also removes gas and digestive secretions, but through a small slit in your stomach rather than through a tube in your nose.

If you have a sore throat after surgery, you're not alone. This is a result of the tube you had inserted through your mouth and into you lungs during surgery. During surgery this tube allowed the machine to do the breathing for you while you were unconscious.

You'll also have another tube, called a catheter, inserted directly into your bladder. This tube drains urine into an external pouch, and allows your healthcare team to monitor your urine output, thus detecting signs of dehydration early on.

What Do I Do about My New Ostomy?

If you had a colostomy or an ileostomy, you don't need to worry too much about taking care of your ostomy immediately after your ostomy surgery. Most colostomy and ileostomy patients don't start taking care of their new additions right away. In fact, many ignore them. They may take a curious peek, but that's about it. During the post-surgery period, your nurses will take over the care of your ostomy for you. Since the digestive system is still resting from ostomy surgery, taking care of the ostomy at this stage mostly means changing the dressing.

Within 24 to 48 hours after surgery, your WOC nurse will fit you with a new appliance, or pouch, for the first time. Your stoma size, as well as your abdominal contour and firmness, will fluctuate for the first few weeks following surgery. For this reason, your WOC nurse will "custom cut" or "cut to fit" the opening on each new pouch during this period. After about six weeks, when your stoma size has settled down, you'll probably be able to use pre-sized systems available from suppliers like Convatec and Hollister. (For more about basic ostomy care and appliances, see chapter 7.)

Until then, though, you'll have to custom cut the opening on each new pouch. If you aren't able to cut them yourself, due to problems such as manual dexterity or eyesight, ask someone to help you (such as your WOC nurse, a relative or a friend).

If you had a urostomy, however, you can't take the "I'll just ignore it except for a quick peek" approach because urine flow starts right after the urostomy is created and remains constant from then on. In fact, if urine flow isn't constant, it's a sign that something's wrong, and you should notify your doctor immediately. Because your urostomy is active from the moment it's created, you'll need to learn more about caring for it more quickly than people with new colostomies or ileostomies. Your nurse will provide you with all the help you need to start caring for your urostomy.

If the rectum is removed as part of colostomy or ileostomy surgery, you'll notice a rather tender wound in the sensitive perineal area. The perineal area, or perineum, is the area between the genitals and where the anus once was. This area needs to be cared for with dressing changes and, possibly, sitz baths.

Beginning to Care for Your Ostomy

Soon, though, your healthcare team will begin to provide you with instructions on how to care for your ostomy. Your WOC nurse will provide you with instructions on how to apply and empty the pouch, clean the stoma, and take care of the skin around the stoma. If you have a colostomy, you may also receive instruction in colostomy irrigation. There are several choices when caring for your ostomy, depending in part on what kind of ostomy you have. Your nurse should discuss your options with you. Ultimately, though, how you choose to care for your ostomy is up to you. Basic ostomy care instructions are also provided in chapter 5.

Often, patients find they receive instruction on how to care for their new ostomy in the days after surgery when they're still tired, in pain, and on a morphine drip. As a result, they don't fully absorb them. Most nurses know this, and are willing to repeat the lessons – even after you've returned home. Let your WOC nurse know that you may need more instruction after you have left the hospital.

Don, 48, the new owner of a colostomy, comments:

A week after I went home from the hospital, I visited an enterostomal therapy (ET) nurse who gave me another lesson on colostomy care. He also gave me several products to try. I discovered one company's pouch worked well for me, and I had no problems after that.

Post-Surgery Homeopathy and Aromatherapy

Homeopathy

In the last chapter, we looked at homeopathic medicines that are useful before surgery. Homeopathic medicines can also be useful after surgery. We'll investigate a few of those in this section.

Keep in mind that the length of time of treatment can and should be different for everyone, depending upon the intensity of symptoms. You should take the recommended dose as long as your pain persists but, in general, don't take them for more than a couple of days. If you're not sure, consult a homeopath or other health professional trained in homeopathy. (And always mention homeopathic medicine to your surgeon.) So, for post-surgery care, take a look at the following:

- Directly after surgery, homeopaths recommend that you take two doses of *Arnica* (6, 12 or 30 – the ingestible form, not the topical ointment) homeopathic remedy, with one hour between the two doses.
- *Bellis perennis* is often recommended by homeopaths for after abdominal surgery when deep internal tissue has been affected (as it has in ostomy surgery). Take from two to eight doses of *Bellis perennis* (6 or 30) over a two-day period following your surgery.
- After abdominal surgery, you may experience gas, or have a distended abdomen without being able to release gas. *Raphanus* (6 or 30) is a common remedy for people who have a distended abdomen but are unable to expel gas. On the other hand, if your abdominal area is more painful than distended, you may want to try *Colocynthis* (6 or 30). Take either remedy every two hours during intense pain and every four hours during mild discomfort. In all cases, if improvement is not obvious after 24 hours, consider another remedy.

Aromatherapy

If you're feeling stressed and anxious after surgery (and you're not alone if you are), you can try the relaxing aromatherapy massage formula mentioned in the pre-surgery aromatherapy section on page 51. If you're also experiencing the fatigue that's common after ostomy surgery, try the following aromatherapy blend, made from oils known for their stimulating and enlivening effect on the body and mind:

- Combine 6 drops of bergamot oil, 2 drops of lemon oil, 2 drops of eucalyptus oil, 1 drop of cinnamon oil, and 1 drop of peppermint oil to 2 ounces of vegetable oil (canola and grapeseed oils from the grocery store are also fine). Use this as a massage or after-bath body oil, but avoid applying it directly to the stoma, the incision, or the skin around it.

Other oils known for their invigorating effect are clary sage, spruce, pine, and rosemary. Again, you can dilute any of these in two ounces of vegetable oil.

If you don't have the energy to make up massage oil, just put a couple of drops of any of these oils on a tissue, and inhale deeply. You can also add a drop or two of any of these oils to an aromatherapy diffuser, light bulb ring, or simply a bowl of hot water to diffuse them into your home. Aromatherapy diffusers and light bulb rings are available from many health food stores.

Bladder Infections

If you had a colostomy or ileostomy, you probably wore a bladder catheter to drain urine into an external pouch after surgery. Unfortunately, some people experience bladder infections after wearing a catheter. Symptoms of a bladder infection include a constant need to urinate and a burning sensation when you do. If you have a bladder infection, the usual treatment is antibiotics and lots of fluids. Cranberry juice, in particular, contains substances that help prevent bacteria from adhering to the walls of the bladder. Since bacteria in the bladder is what causes bladder infections, cranberry juice can be helpful in both prevention and healing.

In fact, if your bladder infection is mild, you may want to try cranberry juice as a first line of defense. Drink between 10 and 16 ounces of unsweetened cranberry juice per day. Be sure to buy the pure, unsweetened kind – you can find it in health food stores. Be careful, though: the kind you'll see on grocery store shelves is usually mostly grape juice and full of sugar; it contains only a small amount of cranberry juice. Alternatively, if you really can't stand the taste, you can take cranberry in capsule form as well. Take one to two capsules of concentrated cranberry daily.

Another herbal remedy for bladder infections is the following tea, made from herbs reputed to soothe bladder inflammation:

- Combine 1 teaspoon each of marshmallow root and echinacea root, and 1/2 teaspoon of Oregon grape root with 2 cups of water, and simmer for 30 minutes. Drink one cup of the tea two to three times per day.

However, if your infection gets worse or if it's severe to start off with, don't hesitate to see your doctor immediately to obtain antibiotics to get rid of it. If left untreated, bladder infections can develop into serious kidney infections.

Life Goes On

Here are some suggestions to help you recover from ostomy surgery, adapted from an article that appeared on About.com's Inflammatory Bowel Disease website.

1. Remember to take things slow at first. You've been through serious surgery, and both your body and mind need to heal from it. Try to remember that you'll get a little better each day.

2. Express your emotions. Be sad, angry, or just plain depressed if you feel like it. Having ostomy surgery means many changes in your life, and these emotions are natural and normal. Read books and magazines about ostomies (try the The Ostomy Quarterly, a magazine published by the United Ostomy Association). If you're connected to the Internet, go to one of the many websites dedicated to those who've undergone ostomy surgery. Hearing from others who are experiencing the same emotions that you are can help you feel less alone.

3. Keep busy at home – especially if you tend to get bored when you can't get out of the house. Your body will be tired and sore from surgery, and you may have trouble concentrating because of your pain medication. Stock up on good movies, magazines, and easy-to-read books. One woman with a new ostomy claims that reading four Harlequin romances per day kept her fully occupied during the initial healing period!

4. Don't do any lifting (typically no more than five pounds) or heavy housecleaning, especially vacuuming, which is hard on the abdominal muscles. Remember – children, cats, dogs, grocery bags, and laundry baskets count as too heavy! Your doctor will tell you when you're ready to undertake these tasks again. In the meantime, why not take advantage of the situation and let someone else do the chores?

5. Get some light exercise, such as walking, as soon as you can. This

helps the digestive system to get moving again, and gets you out and about, too. Try not to overdo it, though. Your body is still recovering and it needs rest. When you and your doctor feel that you're ready, ease into an exercise program gradually.

6. Don't engage in sex until your doctor says that it's okay. Don't be afraid to ask your healthcare team about when you'll be well enough to have sex – it's a very important question that deserves to be addressed. Your mental and emotional readiness is important too. Discuss how you feel with your partner. Most people report that they "know" when they're ready. So go with what's comfortable.

7. When you go to bed, try putting a pillow between your knees, and holding another against your stomach to increase sleeping comfort. You can also try putting a pillow on your chair for increased comfort.

8. Allow someone to help you deal with day-to-day chores, such as grocery shopping, meal preparation and cleaning. If friends or relatives aren't available, check with the UOA or your local hospital about the availability of volunteers. Even if these organizations don't directly provide these services, they may be able to direct you to a volunteer group that can deliver your medications and groceries, or just come by for a short visit.

5
BASIC OSTOMY CARE

Caring for an ostomy isn't as hard as it used to be. Back before ostomy surgery became relatively common, people used great ingenuity to come up with unique methods of caring for their ostomies. Rubber gloves, cigar cases and even empty tuna fish cans have all been employed as ways to collect ostomy output. Fortunately, you won't have to go to such lengths to take care of your ostomy. The goal of the next two chapters is to help you learn to manage your ostomy, so that it doesn't end up managing you!

This chapter introduces you to the different methods of ostomy care – from *laissez faire* to irrigation. (Keep in mind that some methods may not be available to you because of the type of ostomy you have.) Chapter 6 describes ostomy appliances (also called pouches or pouching systems) in more detail, and answers some of the most common questions about ostomy care.

If It's My Ostomy, Why Do I Feel Like It's Managing Me?

The method you end up using to manage your ostomy should fit your lifestyle and personality as closely as possible. But for the first two or three months after ostomy surgery, it may seem like your ostomy is managing you. That's normal, and it happens for several reasons.

First, your ostomy is probably going to be on its worst behavior during these first few months. Most people's digestive systems take a while to get back to normal, and this means that your ostomy may be a bit temperamental at first. Even if you have a urostomy, it will take your body a while to adjust to the changes in its urinary tract.

Second, you're quite likely still making the adjustments needed to deal with your ostomy – both physically and psychologically.

Abdominal surgery is physically taxing on the body, and you probably won't have the energy you had prior to surgery. (Of course, this depends on why you got your ostomy – if you had surgery as a result of a long battle with severe IBD, you may begin to feel better right from the start.)

Your physical limitations will probably make psychological adjustments necessary, too. Because you now have completely different "plumbing," you'll probably also be experiencing changes in your self-image (see more about this in "Chapter 9: Body image, relationships and sexuality").

As well, just being ill is difficult for many people. You may have been energetic and independent before you got your ostomy, and now you're making a slow (but sure) recovery from major surgery. At first, it will be hard even to make a meal for yourself and wash up afterwards. Being dependent on others for things that you used to do yourself can be difficult psychologically. Rest assured, though, that your energy and independence will return. In fact, many people with ostomies report that once they'd recovered from the effects of surgery, they gained energy and freedom they'd never known before.

All of these factors can make learning to care for your ostomy that much more difficult in the beginning. But learning to effectively care for your ostomy is possible. Millions of people have done it, and so can you!

How you care for your ostomy depends on what type of ostomy you have.

- If you have a colostomy, there are several ways to go about the day-to-day care of your ostomy. Most people use pouching systems, which collect waste and are easy to dispose of. You may choose to irrigate your colostomy – though this option requires manual dexterity and considerable time.
- Ileosotomies require that a pouch be worn at all times, as the stool is quite liquid. The exception is continent ileostomies.– if the continent ileostomy is working properly, pouches are unnecessary.
- For urostomies, on the other hand, urine output is constant. Because of this, conventional urostomies always require use of a pouching system (although, again, continent urostomies do not).

Basic Care for Colostomies and Ileostomies

When you were in the hospital, your WOC nurse probably fitted you with a one-piece, custom-fitted, disposable appliance that was transparent, rather than opaque. These post-surgery pouches are transparent because it's necessary for hospital staff to continually observe the stoma and its output, to ensure that your recovery is happening according to plan. The appliance was custom-fitted to match the size of your stoma, since your stoma will not yet have settled down to its eventual, permanent size. And they're disposable, simply because that's easier to manage at first.

Usually, it's best to continue using a one-piece, disposable, custom-cut appliance for at least the first two months after surgery. Why? Generally, your digestive system – and your ostomy – are somewhat unpredictable in the first few months after surgery. You may also experience weight changes over these first few months as your body adjusts to its new plumbing. For example, many IBD sufferers will experience healthy weight gains as the body is finally able to absorb the nutrients that were previously flushed out by diarrhea. It's usually best to wait until your weight stabilizes and your ostomy settles down before moving on to other methods of ostomy care

If you prefer not to see the contents of the pouch, opaque ones are available. But some people with poor eyesight or with a difficult stoma placement may choose to stay with transparent pouches, finding that they're easier to manage.

Because your ostomy takes a while to settle down after surgery, you'll probably want to use a *laissez faire* approach to caring for your ostomy at first. This means that you'll leave your ostomy to it's own devices: it will produce stool whenever it wants, and you'll need to use a pouching system to collect the stool. So, for the first couple of months at least, you'll be using some type of pouching system.

You'll be relieved to learn that stoma size (and behavior) will settle down about two months after surgery. After about six weeks, you'll probably be able to use pre-sized pouching systems available from ostomy suppliers like Convatec and Hollister. These pouching systems are described on page 72.

Options for Managing Colostomies

After your colostomy settles down and your bowel movements become more predictable, you may decide to stick with the *laissez faire* approach you've been using up until now, in which you use some type of pouching system, or appliance, to collect waste. You may also decide to explore other ways of managing your colostomy. Each ostomy care method described below has its advantages and disadvantages, but what it eventually boils down to is your own personal preference.

Appliances (pouching systems)

At the hospital, you were likely fitted with a two-piece, transparent pouch with a custom-fitted opening. Again, it's best to continue using this type of pouching system for the first couple of months after surgery, because the stoma's size and behavior are still settling down. However, if you decide to use a pouching system to care for your ostomy over the long term, you'll probably want to make appliance adjustments to increase ease of use. We'll look at all your appliance options in chapter 6.

In fact, after exploring alternatives like dietary control and colostomy irrigation, many people find that they like the convenience of a pouching system best of all. After all, although "pouch skills" take practice to perfect, they're not particularly difficult to learn. Pouches are comfortable, odor-free, invisible under clothing, and made from "rustle-free" plastic so that they're soundless when you move.

Colostomy irrigation

Another method of ostomy care that doesn't require that you use a pouching system is irrigation. Again, this method is an option only for those with a colostomy with fully formed output, such as a sigmoid or descending colostomy. It also tends to work better for those who had regular bowel habits before surgery.

What is irrigation? Instead of wearing a pouch to collect colostomy output, you use special colostomy irrigation equipment (available from ostomy appliance suppliers) to evacuate the stool into the toilet while you relax on the toilet seat. It's similar to a self-conducted enema that keeps the bowel stool-free for up to 72 hours (although most people find that 24 to 48 hours is the norm).

Ideally, there's no stool output between irrigations, because the bowel is flushed completely clean. Between irrigations, many people wear a small piece of absorbent dressing. For more security, you may also choose to use a small, compact "security pouch" that collects stool drainage between irrigations, if any occurs.

Sounds pretty good, doesn't it?

But the catch is that irrigation can take up to an hour (and sometimes more, at the beginning) because it takes time to coax the stool from the bowel. The good news is that this time requirement diminishes as your technique improves. And the more relaxed you are, the more the bowel seems to cooperate. Once you're familiar with the technique and you're relaxed and comfortable, irrigating your colostomy can take as little as 30 minutes. Some people even look forward to this piece of personal time!

Correct irrigation technique, as well as sufficient time, is crucial to make this method effective. In general, to irrigate your colostomy, you must:

- Obtain a colostomy irrigation set from an ostomy appliance supplier.
- Have uninterrupted use of a bathroom and toilet for at least one hour per day (at least at first).
- Have patience, patience, and more patience!

Whether you decide to irrigate your colostomy or not is your choice. Irrigation doesn't work for everyone. In fact, some people find it disagreeable, time-consuming, or ineffective (they pass stool through the stoma anyway, despite having irrigated). Some people have lifestyles that don't allow them to irrigate at a predetermined time each day. Others don't have the amount of uninterrupted bathroom time required for a successful irrigation.

In general, if irrigation is not accomplishing continence, or if it's making you uncomfortable, you should not be doing it. The choice to irrigate or not to irrigate is up to you.

If you decide to irrigate, consult your doctor first to ensure that it's a good option for you. It's also best to consult a WOC nurse before attempting irrigation, to get guidance on how to do it.

Dietary control

It's a rare ostomy that can be managed through dietary control alone. However, if your bowels were *very* regular prior to surgery, you may be able to encourage this regularity after surgery through diet.

Certain foods stimulate stool production; others inhibit it. Some people are able to control ostomy output by making use of this fact. They eat at regular intervals, and restrict themselves to certain foods. This lets them train their ostomies to produce stool only at regular intervals – for example, every morning after breakfast. When they expect a bowel movement, they simply attach a pouch, and remove it when the movement is complete. The rest of the time, they simply cover the ostomy with a pad or – for more security – a small pouch, in case of accidents.

This type of colostomy management is appropriate only if your ostomy produces fully formed output, such as a sigmoid or descending colostomy. Less formed output, like that produced by an ascending colostomy, just cannot be regulated in this way, and is more likely to be released at unpredictable intervals or continuously.

Keep in mind that you're more likely to be able to control your ostomy with diet if your bowel movements were extremely regular before ostomy surgery, and this just isn't the case for many people.

The colostomy plug

Because it allows you to regulate the bowel, irrigation is sometimes referred to as a continent ostomy management procedure. But another type of continent colostomy care method may be available to you, as well.

This is a device that acts as an artificial sphincter, restoring control over the evacuation of bowel waste and eliminating the need for a pouch. The device, a lubricated "stoma plug," is inserted into the colostomy to seal it off. The stoma plug looks similar to a small tampon, and has a plastic cap at the base.

While the stoma plug may take some getting used to, it does have several advantages. You can wear it for up to twelve hours at a time and remain continent throughout that time, without the need for a pouch or daily irrigation. When the plug is removed, the build-up of stool behind it is evacuated into a pouch, or, with practice, into the toilet.

A new plug is needed with each wear, however, since the original plug cannot be re-inserted into the colostomy.

This method of colostomy management can be difficult to learn, making help from a WOC nurse critical. If you're interested in a continent colostomy, speak to your doctor or WOC nurse first. This is important, because these methods aren't recommended for everyone. For example, it may not be appropriate for you if you suffered from an inflammatory bowel disease.

Generally, it's an option for people who have a sigmoid or descending colostomy that produces well-formed stool four times a day or less. The stoma should have a diameter of 3/4 of an inch to 2 inches, and it shouldn't protrude more than 1 inch from the abdomen.

Options for Managing Ileostomies

If you have an ileostomy, keep in mind that – even after an adjustment period – it'll likely be less predictable than a colostomy. You probably didn't have regular bowel movements prior to surgery due to IBD, so it'll be more difficult for you to regulate your digestive system now. Also, because an ileostomy is located further up in the GI tract, the output is less formed and, therefore, less easy to regulate. For these reasons, all people with conventional Brooke ileostomies rely on appliances or pouching systems to care for their ostomies. Unlike colostomies, ileostomies aren't responsive to efforts to regulate them through diet, and they can't be managed using irrigation.

Continent ileostomies

Continent ileostomies present another set of self-care challenges. A common problem for people with intestinal or ileoanal pouches is pouchitis (inflammation of the lining of the pouch), which is usually cleared up with antibiotics.

The appliances you need to manage your continent ileostomy depend in part on whether you have a stoma or not. If you have a continent intestinal reservoir, you must drain the intestinal reservoir using a catheter. However, if you have an ileoanal reservoir, you will not be using any equipment at all – you'll be able to control your bowel movements, although your stool will be quite loose and frequent, especially at the beginning.

Basic Care for Urostomies

Right after surgery, your new urostomy pouch will be hooked up to a bedside receptacle. Soon after surgery, though, you'll need to learn how to attach, remove, and empty the pouch yourself.

Like post-surgery ileostomy and colostomy appliances, your urostomy pouch will be clear, rather than opaque, so that medical staff can ensure that your urostomy is functioning correctly. It'll also be custom-cut to fit your stoma, since stoma size will vary at first until the stoma settles down to its eventual size.

Unless your urostomy is continent, your urostomy care process will include a pouching system, worn during the day, as well as some type of night drainage system. The goal of night drainage systems is to increase the appliance's storage capacity, and prevent you from having to get up and empty the pouch every two to three hours throughout the night. Night drainage systems can include either a bedside receptacle or a "night pouch" that's larger than your regular ostomy pouch.

Larger capacity urostomy pouches are also available for special situations, such as traveling, in which the appliance cannot be emptied as frequently as normal. For example, a special leg bag can be connected to the pouch by tubing and worn under the clothes. This allows for extra storage space. It's especially good for airplane or car trips when rest stops are infrequent. Urostomy pouches also include a non-reflux valve, which prevents urine from "backing up" into the kidneys, and prevents leakage, especially when you're lying down.

You should empty the pouch when it's about one-third full of urine. This prevents the pouch from getting too full and pulling off. It also prevents the possibility of urine flowing backward into the kidneys, which can lead to a serious kidney infection.

Typically, you'll need to change your pouch every four to seven days, or when any of the following occur: leakage, unusual itching under the pouch, or burning under the pouch. If any of these symptoms do occur, remove the pouch and examine the stoma and the skin around it. If the symptoms persist, don't hesitate to make an appointment with your WOC nurse.

If you have a continent urostomy, you don't need to wear an appliance. Care of continent urostomies involves draining the internal pouch using a catheter four to six times per day. As with other types of continent procedures, problems like pouchitis are possible. If you experience problems with your continent urostomy, consult your WOC nurse.

6
SELECTING AN APPLIANCE

There are all sorts of ostomy appliances (also called pouching systems) available. In fact, there are so many choices that there's absolutely no reason for you to make do with an ill fitting, uncomfortable, or inconvenient appliance. While it's true that finding the right appliance might take some trial and error, there are ample resources for you to turn to in your search. WOC nurses are a great resource, and should be your main source of information. It's your WOC nurse's job to make sure that your ostomy is as easy for you to manage as possible. Customer service representatives for ostomy suppliers like Convatec can be very helpful in educating you about what's available. There are also many websites that provide information about how to use pouching systems, as well as discussion groups where people help each other solve both internal and external pouch-related problems. Many of these resources are listed at the end of this book.

About Appliances

During the post-surgery recovery period, you were probably fitted with a two-piece, clear appliance, so that the hospital staff could ensure that your ostomy was functioning properly. This two-piece appliance also probably had a starter hole that was custom-cut to fit your stoma, allowing for changes in stoma size as the ostomy settled down after surgery. The appliance was probably closed-end, meaning that it couldn't be emptied. After the stoma produced feces, the nurse removed and disposed of it, and attached a new one. Closed-end appliances are usually suitable when ostomy size and behavior are still settling down, but they may not be the most convenient for long term use.

So what type of appliance is best for long term use? Well, that depends on the type of ostomy you have, and on your personal preferences. This chapter provides a basic overview of the different choices available to you, but – again – the best resource for determining the most suitable option for you is your WOC nurse.

Anatomy of an Appliance

An ostomy appliance is made up of two components: a skin adhesive barrier wafer and a pouch. You'll have the choice of a one-piece or two-piece appliance. Both one-piece and two-piece appliances can be either closed-end or drainable.

What's the difference between one- and two-piece appliances? In a one-piece appliance, the two components (skin adhesive barrier wafer and pouch) are joined together, and are applied together to the skin in a one-step procedure. By contrast, each of the two components of a two-piece appliance is applied separately in a two-step procedure. The skin adhesive barrier wafer has a plastic flange material attached to it. This wafer is applied to the body first. The pouch also has a plastic flange material attached to it; to complete the application process, you attach it to the flange on the wafer.

Both one-piece and two-piece pouches can be drainable or closed-end, depending on your needs and preferences. Drainable pouches can be emptied as often as needed. Closed-end pouches are disposed of once they're full.

Both one-piece and two-piece pouching systems can be either opaque or transparent, and often have a fiber or net backing on the side that touches the body to help absorb perspiration and increase comfort. Unlike the cumbersome ostomy gear of yesteryear, all contemporary appliances are made from very lightweight material, and are designed to be easy-to-use and odor-free. Suppliers often offer smaller sizes of each pouching product; these are convenient for use during sports and sex. Most ostomy appliances in use today are disposable, which means that they are used just once, then thrown away.

If you have a urostomy, you'll want to use an appliance specifically designed for urostomies. Urostomy appliances have a drainage valve or spout at the end – this makes them easy to empty. That's a good thing, because urine constantly collects in the pouch and must be drained frequently. All urostomy pouches are constructed with a watertight valve at the bottom; opening the valve and releasing the collected urine into the toilet empties them.

In addition to consulting your WOC nurse, one of the best ways to get an idea of your appliance options is to contact the customer service department of one of the larger ostomy appliance suppliers and ask them what they offer.

Convexity in Pouching Systems

When choosing a pouching system, convexity is another issue to consider. Convexity is the outward (convex) curving of the portion of the pouch that has contact with the skin. If the skin around your stoma is irritated, it may be because the stoma is short, flush with the skin, or retracted. These types of stomas can cause problems with standard pouching systems. Appliances that incorporate convexity address this problem. The portion of the pouch that has contact with the skin (usually the skin barrier) curves firmly against the skin, encouraging the stoma to protrude slightly, creating a very tight seal on the peristomal skin.

Appliance Accessories

Other appliance accessories are important to help ensure that your pouching system works well for you. Your WOC nurse is a good source of information about these products. You can also contact an ostomy supplier for more information; they'll be happy to provide you with samples.

Here's a brief overview of the difference accessories you may need:

- Protective skin barrier creams, lotions and powders prepare the skin for the application of the barrier.
- Skin cleansers make cleaning the skin around the stoma easy. They're designed not to leave any residue, which can interfere with the seal of the adhesive.
- Deodorants help control odor from the pouch, and are available as either drops or sprays. Colostomy pouches often have built-in odor filters, whereas urostomy and ileostomy pouches generally do not.
- Adhesives secure the appliance to the skin when you're putting on an appliance, and adhesive removers help remove the appliance from the skin and minimize skin irritation. The latter is often packaged in individual wipes, which are convenient when changing the appliance.
- Pouch covers cover the pouch. Many people prefer to use them because they feel better against the skin.

- Clamps or clips are used to secure the end of a drainable pouch until it's time to empty it.
- Belts gently bind the pouch to your body. They're available in different sizes to fit every body. Some people prefer to wear belts when swimming or enjoying sports or sex, so that the pouch is secured to the body.

Ostomy Care Q & A

How do I control odor and gas?

Ostomy appliances usually include charcoal filters to control odor, and valves that let you release gas at convenient moments (such as when you're in the bathroom), thereby avoiding the appliance blowing up like a balloon. As well, you can purchase deodorant tablets that are ingested, or placed in the pouch itself. You can also adjust your diet to minimize odor and gas. Chapter 5 includes more information about managing your diet.

How often should I empty the appliance?

The answer depends on what type of ostomy you have and on the amount of output. In general, most types of ostomy appliances (including urostomy appliances) should be emptied several times a day, or when they're one-third to one-half full. Regular emptying reduces the possibility of leakage and prevents uncomfortable bulkiness under clothing. If you have a closed-end appliance, you'll simply remove it and dispose of it. If you have a drainable appliance, you can empty it into the toilet, then reseal the tail with a clamp.

How do I empty the appliance?

To empty the appliance, sit on the toilet with the pouch between your legs, leaning forward. With the enclosure clamp on, turn the contents upward away from the body. Remove the clamp carefully (or, if you have a urostomy, release the spout), aim the end of the pouch into the toilet and empty it. If you're emptying a urostomy appliance, make sure all urine has drained completely off the inside of the spout so that no urine gets on your clothes. Otherwise, wipe off the end of the appliance with toilet paper. If you wish, you can add a splash of mouthwash to help control odor. Refasten with the clamp, folding it once. Don't fold the end of the pouch more than once, since this can cause leakage.

Remember to place the clamp out of the way when you're emptying your pouch. Always carry a spare pouch clamp with you when you will be emptying away from home or are traveling. Take your time when refastening the pouch clamp as you may be more apt to drop the clip into the toilet when you're in a hurry.

How often should I change the appliance?

Like emptying frequency, the frequency with which you change your pouch depends on your ostomy, the type of output, your activities and your own preference.

For example, sports enthusiasts may need to change appliances more frequently than those who are less active, since the high level of physical activity places more stress on the appliance's seal.

Likewise, if the output of your stoma is liquid or caustic (as it can be with ileostomies), the skin barrier may break down more quickly. This means you'll probably need to change your appliance more often. You may also want to investigate appliances and accessories specifically designed to manage more caustic stoma output, such as ultra-durable skin barriers. Check with your ostomy supplier for more information. Many offer free samples for you to try.

How do I change the appliance?

Most people develop a routine for changing the appliance. Here are some basic guidelines to help you get started. Generally, the best time to change your pouch is first thing in the morning (your stoma will be less active before you've had anything to eat or drink).

- Prepare as much of your pouching system as you can. For example, cut the skin barrier, remove paper backing from skin barrier, and apply paste to the back of skin barrier. Make sure your clothing is out of the way.
- If your appliance is drainable, empty it into the toilet. If it's disposable, place it in a plastic bag and put it in the garbage receptacle.
- Remove your pouch carefully working from the top down, supporting the skin. Try not to rip the adhesive from the skin.
- Clean the skin around the stoma with warm water and a moistened wipes (wipes are available from ostomy suppliers). It may help to use a dry wipe first to remove any residue and mucous from the base of the stoma. If you wish to use plain soap (no fragrance, oils or other

additives) you can do so, but it's not necessary. Any soap, such as ostomy soap, must be washed off before drying. Avoid direct contact with stool.

- Dry your skin thoroughly with a dry towelette. Don't worry if your stoma bleeds slightly when washed. This is normal. If you notice lots of blood, however, consult your WOC nurse.
- Apply skin protection as required (such as skin protecting creams, lotions or powders).
- Remove the appliance-backing paper and position the appliance carefully and slowly (it may be easier to do this standing upright). Use a mirror to help you see your stoma.
- Once it is in place, ensure that the wafer is smooth and stuck firmly to the skin, paying particular attention to the base. If you're using two-piece pouching system, apply the pouch to the wafer.

How do I dispose of the appliance?

Never flush your appliance down the toilet. (Some pouches contain liners that are designed to be flushable; if you have one of these, remove it and flush it down the toilet.) Empty the contents of your pouch into the toilet. If you use a drainable appliance, set the clamp aside before disposing of the appliance. Wrap the used appliance in a plastic bag and put it in the garbage. Some appliances are actually packaged in a bag that can be used for disposal.

How do I make sure my pouch fits properly?

As mentioned earlier, any weight gains or losses will require that you revise your pouching strategy. Weight change is particularly likely in the months directly following ostomy surgery. You'll need to re-measure the stoma and re-size the appliance to fit it. For example, sore peristomal skin can occur soon after surgery if the wafer of the appliance is cut too large, allowing stool to make contact with the skin. This can be very painful, particularly if the stool is less formed and more caustic.

If you're having trouble with leakage, consult with your WOC nurse to find out how to improve pouch fit. Consider visiting your WOC nurse two to three times per year to reassess pouching methods and to assess problems.

How much does an appliance cost?

Cost varies, depending on the type of appliance you decide to use. Insurance covers part of the cost of ostomy supplies for some people;

check with your insurance company to find out if this is the case for you. Your WOC nurse may also be able to give you guidance about cost.

What if I have problems with my appliance?

If you are having trouble with your appliance, arrange a meeting with your WOC nurse. He or she is in the best position to diagnose your problem and suggest solutions.

You can also try contacting the Customer Service department of ostomy supply companies such as Hollister and Convatec. Contact information for these companies is provided at the end of this book. They should be able to suggest products that address your problems, and most make free samples available for you to try. With help from a WOC nurse – and perhaps a bit of trial and error – you should be able to get things working smoothly.

Problems may include odor, a noisy pouch that rustles when you move, or an ill-fitting appliance. The latter can cause both leakage and irritated skin around the stoma. It can also be a factor in odor control.

How do I recognize problems with my ostomy?

The stoma should be moist, and red or pink – much like the inside of your mouth. It may bleed slightly on contact, but the skin around it should be free of lesions, inflammation, encrustation, or ulcers. In short, it should look like the rest of your skin. If the stoma swells or turns purple, black, or white, contact your WOC nurse or doctor immediately, or go to the emergency room for evaluation.

A word about bleeding: it's normal for the stoma to bleed, because of its high concentration of blood vessels. If your stoma bleeds a lot, apply pressure with a dry cloth for ten minutes. If the bleeding doesn't stop, or if it occurs frequently, contact your WOC nurse or go to the emergency room for evaluation. Keep in mind that some medications may contribute to bleeding, such as Aspirin, Coumadin, and Ticlid.

The most common types of problems tend to be skin problems, such as injury and infection; or disease-related skin conditions, such as dermatitis, caused by an allergy to pouching products.

If you notice any problems with the skin around your stoma, contact your WOC nurse as soon as possible. Your WOC nurse is trained to help you identify, and manage and prevent problems with your ostomy.

7
DIET, SKIN CARE AND MEDICATION

Do you believe you'll need to follow a strict diet now that you have an ostomy? Are you concerned about how to care for the skin around your stoma? Are you worried about whether your medication is being absorbed properly now that you have an ostomy?

If so, you're not alone. Diet, skin care and medication are three of the most common concerns of people with new ostomies.

As far as diet is concerned, it's just not true that you need to follow a special diet now that you have an ostomy. However, the foods that bothered you before your ostomy surgery will probably continue to do so. And if you had to follow a special diet for any other health condition (such as diabetes), you will need to continue to follow it. Your goal is to create a varied, enjoyable diet that adds to your quality of life rather than causing problems for you and your ostomy. This chapter provides some suggestions on how to do that.

If you're worried about caring for the skin around your stoma, this chapter should help put your fears to rest. Most people have few problems, and if problems do occur, they're usually minor and easily handled. We'll look at how to prevent and manage different skin problems, and how to know when to consult your doctor or WOC nurse.

And if you're wondering how medication will work with your ostomy, then this chapter is for you. In general, you don't need to make many (if any) changes if you have a colostomy or a urostomy. If you have an ileostomy, though, you may need to be a bit more careful.

Dietary Guidelines and Nutrition

The first thing to remember is that an ostomy doesn't, by itself, restrict you from eating any particular foods. One exception is if you've had most or all of your large intestine removed. In this case, you may experience problems with certain foods that are hard to digest. You're better off using caution when eating foods high in fiber, such as raw vegetables, popcorn and nuts. That's because if these foods aren't completely chewed, they may cause "blockage," or intestinal obstruction, at the stoma opening. Most foods don't cause problems if they're chewed well, though. Although blockage is usually treatable at home, it can mean a trip to the hospital in more severe cases. All in all, it's probably best to take a preventative approach and be careful with hard-to-digest foods. We'll look at a more complete list of these a bit later, along with some precautions to take when eating them.

If you have any other health conditions, such as diabetes, remember that you still need to avoid foods that aggravate them. Likewise, if certain foods bothered you before you got your ostomy, they'll probably still do so. However, if you really enjoy a particular food, it may be worth experimenting with it. Add it back to your diet, and pay attention to the effect it has on your digestive system and on the way you feel. You may find that some foods that previously irritated your digestive system aren't a problem anymore.

Although having an ostomy doesn't doom you forever to a bland and boring diet, there are certain guidelines that you should follow with respect to nutrition. For the most part, these guidelines are the basis of any healthy diet, and everyone should be following them – not just people with ostomies!

If you've got an ileostomy (either conventional or continent), the fact that you no longer have a large intestine means that you have to be more vigilant about dehydration. One of the functions of the colon is to absorb fluid and salt, and now that yours is gone, you need to be sure to ingest lots of fluids, vitamins and minerals. This is particularly true when you're exercising vigorously and in hot weather.

Basic Dietary Guidelines

While an ostomy itself doesn't necessarily require a change in diet, it does provide a good opportunity for you to evaluate your diet and create a diet that works for you. Your goal is to support your physical health, including but not limited to your ostomy, and to enjoy your diet as much as possible. Most hospitals employ one or more dieticians. Ideally, you should take this opportunity to sit down with one of them and work out a diet that suits your particular needs. The dietician should be able to provide you with guidelines about how to obtain sufficient nutrients from the food you eat, as well as special information that will help you take care of concerns you may have with your ostomy (such as odor and gas). The dietician should also take into account your history: what has your diet been like in the past, and how will it change now that you have an ostomy. You should also be informed about how the foods you eat will affect your stoma's output – for example, which foods are more likely to cause odor. To some extent, this is a trial and error process.

Tim, 25, who has a J- pouch, learned to manage his diet this way:

> Four weeks after surgery, my WOC nurse told me to follow a regular diet, but I found that some of the things I used to be able to eat now seemed to bother me. So, every time I added a new food to my diet, I kept a food diary to help figure out which foods were irritating to my digestive system and causing diarrhea. After about two weeks of doing this, a pattern became clear. I learned that coffee, fried foods, spicy foods and sweets were causing problems for me.

Here are some basic guidelines that will keep you and your ostomy on good terms.

- Eat regularly. The first few days after you start eating following surgery, you may feel more comfortable eating small, frequent "mini-meals," but after this initial period, it's best to eat three regular meals per day.
- Avoid undereating. Besides compromising your health and depleting your energy, it causes excess gas.
- Chew your food well. Although everyone should chew food well to optimize the body's ability to extract nutrients from food, it is especially important for people with ileostomies to chew food very well. Inadequately chewed food often doesn't digest completely, and can cause blockage at the stoma site.
- Eat a balanced diet. This increases your general health and vitality level. Most countries have general food guidelines that tell you how much of certain foods you should be getting. Follow these guidelines as closely as you can, making use of substitutes as you feel them to be necessary. For example, you may decide to drink soya milk forti-

fied with calcium if milk and other dairy products irritate your digestive system.

- Include lots of dietary fiber in your diet. Eating fiber makes regular,
  formed bowel movements more likely, making it easier for you to
  manage your ostomy – and keeping your digestive system in good
  shape. This is especially important if you are prone to diarrhea. If you
  experience constipation, on the other hand, you may want to limit
  your fiber intake until the problem clears up. See the suggestions in
  the "Dietary Q & A" section later in this chapter.

- Try new foods one at a time. This lets you pinpoint the foods that
  cause problems for you, such as excess gas, constipation, loose stools
  and odor. If you find that a new food is causing problems but you
  don't want to remove it from your diet permanently, eliminate it from
  your diet for a few weeks, then try it again to see if it causes problems.
  It's always possible that something else was causing the problem.

- Try to limit the foods that irritate your digestive system. If you find
  that certain foods always cause problems for you, try to limit them.
  Keep things in perspective, though. Most of us find that even foods
  that are problematic are still worth eating once in a while if we really enjoy them. For example, you may be willing to put up with a bit
  of gas just for the pleasure of indulging in that big bowl of chocolate
  ice cream!

- Try to maintain a constant weight. If you got your ostomy because of
  IBD, you may need to gain weight after ostomy surgery because you
  were underweight before. But once you reach your normal weight, try
  to avoid gaining excess weight. It's not good for your ostomy and can
  cause health problems for you in general. If you want to lose weight,
  do it in a slow, healthy way. Avoid crash diets – they'll cause abrupt
  changes in ostomy size and endanger your health as well. If you feel
  you need to lose or gain weight to reach your optimal health, consider seeing a dietician. Most hospitals have one on staff, and if they
  don't, your doctor or WOC nurse can recommend one.

Dietary Q & A

What is Blockage and How Do I Prevent It?

It's common knowledge that high-fiber foods are good for you. In general, this is true, and your diet should include them. But some types of fibrous foods are particularly hard to digest, and may result in blockage. Blockage, or intestinal obstruction, results when an incompletely digested piece of food fails to exit the body properly through the stoma. Blockages can occur anywhere in the intestinal tract.

Blockage is more likely to occur if you have an ileostomy, since an ileostomy stoma is generally smaller than that of a colostomy because it's made from the ileum rather than the colon.

Blockage can be an emergency, because you can become dehydrated very quickly, and it can be painful if left untreated. Most people never experience a blockage, but it's best to be familiar with the signs of one just in case you do:

- You'll see an almost constant spurting of watery stool.
- You may have abdominal cramping and bloating.
- You may be unable to pass gas or be constipated.
- The stoma or the skin around it may be swollen.
- The stool may have a very strong odor.
- If the blockage is not cleared, the flow of stool will stop, and you'll experience pain and eventually nausea and vomiting.

What should you do if you begin to experience a blockage? Here are some suggestions:

- Don't eat any solid food, and don't take laxatives or stool softeners.
- Try applying a pouch with a larger opening – this provides more room for the stoma to pass the particular food that's blocking it.
- Massage your abdomen gently with your palms. You may want to create an aromatherapy massage oil using essential oils known to relieve indigestion. To do this, combine 12 drops of peppermint oil, 12 drops of sweet orange oil, 8 drops of ginger oil and 5 drops of fennel oil to 4 ounces of vegetable oil. Massage the oil onto your abdomen gently, avoiding direct contact with the stoma and the skin directly around it.
- Try taking a warm bath or shower. A gentle abdominal massage, in combination with the heat of the water, can help soothe and relax you, and release the blockage.

- Try sipping a soothing tea made from ginger, peppermint, chamomile or fennel. Health food stores often offer ready-made "digestive" teas as well. These teas can ease your digestive system and reduce discomfort.

You may be able to clear a relatively slight blockage that lasts less than two hours by following these recommendations. But if your symptoms last more than two or three hours, or if you're nauseous or vomiting, contact your doctor or go to an emergency room immediately.

The best way to prevent blockage is to chew your food well – at least 20 to 25 times. You should also drink lots of water – eight to twelve cups per day.

Eat small amounts of potentially problematic foods, or, if they cause problems for you, avoid them altogether. Here's a list of foods that aren't completely digestible, and therefore may cause problems:

- Celery
- Popcorn
- Chinese vegetables
- Coconut
- Raw pineapple
- Coleslaw
- Raisins and dates (and other dried fruits)
- Nuts and seeds
- Peas
- Vegetable skins
- Mushrooms
- Salads
- Relishes

Don't worry if your abdomen feels sensitive following a blockage – some soreness is normal, and it'll pass. You may want to follow a low-fiber diet for a couple of days following the blockage to give your intestine a chance to rest.

How Do I Reduce Odor With Diet?

Odor results from the digestive process. It's normal to be worried about it (many people are). But if you're following the ostomy care guidelines provided in the previous chapter, it's unlikely that your ostomy is creating a noticeable or problematic odor. Many people are overly conscientious about ostomy odor – especially those with new ostomies. In reality, it's unlikely that odor will be a problem. For one thing, some appliances have odor-resistant filters built right into them. Check with your ostomy supplier to see if they offer one that meets your needs.

If you're worried about odor occurring when you're emptying or changing pouches (especially in public bathrooms), keep a small can of deodorant or a matchbook with you just in case. Some people like to place a teaspoon or so of mouthwash or hydrogen peroxide in the pouch each time they empty it, finding that this neutralizes odor. You may also want to check if it's time to change the pouch – sometimes odor can result if mucus builds up around the stoma.

However, if you do experience problems with odor, it could be your diet that's the culprit. Some foods are particularly likely to cause odor as they're being digested. Luckily, it's usually easy to manage any problems with odor by making changes in the diet. You can remove items that you think are causing problems, and add foods that are known to reduce odor. Here's a list of some foods that are particularly likely to cause odor:

- Alcohol
- Cauliflower
- Asparagus (especially responsible for odor in the urine)
- Fish
- Brussels sprouts
- Cheese
- Baked beans
- Eggs
- Broccoli
- Onions
- Cabbage

Before removing nutritious and favorite foods from your diet permanently, it's important that you experiment to determine whether these foods really are responsible for odor problems. For example, if you experience a problem with a certain food, you might try removing it from your diet temporarily – perhaps for a few weeks. Then add it back, and observe the results.

You may also want to add foods to your diet that are known to reduce odor. For example:

- Yogurt and buttermilk improve the digestive process because of the large amounts of "good" bacteria they contain.
- Some people find that drinking tomato juice and vegetable juice (such as V8) helps control odor.

- In addition to eating lots of yogurt and other acidophilus-containing foods, you may want to consider adding acidophilus supplements to your diet. Studies have shown acidophilus may aid in digestion and improve the absorption of nutrients. Other studies have shown that the ingestion of acidophilus reduces the concentration of enzymes in the stool that promote the formation of carcinogens (cancer-causing agents) in the colon, although it's not yet known whether this can help prevent colon cancer.
- Parsley also helps control stool odor – you can add it as a garnish to your fish, for example, to help mitigate any odor caused by the fish.
- Chlorophyll has been called a natural internal deodorant. It has been used to eliminate bad breath and reduce urine and stool odor. You can obtain chlorophyll from your diet, or you may decide to buy a product containing concentrated chlorophyll. Dietary sources of chlorophyll include dark leafy green vegetables, wheat grass, spirulina, algae, barley grass and chlorella. Since it may be difficult to find some of these items (let alone ingest enough of them to eliminate odor) you may also choose to obtain a prepared product containing concentrated chlorophyll. These powders are usually prepared from the dehydrated juice extracted from vegetables and plants, and are marketed under names like Greens Plus and Green Stuff. You can also obtain chlorophyll in liquid form – check your local health food store.

How much chlorophyll should you take? To reduce odor, take 100 milligrams of chlorophyll twice or three times daily. Start with twice daily; if this doesn't produce results, then increase you intake to three times daily.

How Do I Reduce Gas With Diet?

Some amount of gas production is normal during the digestive process – and everybody releases it (even in public!). Unfortunately, if you have an ostomy, you can't control when it's released. And if you wear a pouch, it can puff out like a balloon if it fills with gas – a very uncomfortable experience. Many ostomy appliances have release valves that let you release gas from the pouch at more opportune moments (such as when you're in the bathroom).

If you're finding gas is a problem, there are a number of things you can do to minimize it.

1. Avoid talking when eating, eating quickly, chewing gum, and drinking through a straw. All of these activities increase the amount of air you swallow, which leads to – you guessed it – more gas.

2. Eat regularly – if you skip meals, your digestive system produces digestive enzymes even though there's nothing to digest. This leads to more gas.

3. Make changes to your diet to minimize or eliminate gas-producing foods. However, as with eliminating odor-producing foods, take care not to permanently remove foods that you love or that are nutritious. Again, you might try removing them for a few weeks, then adding them back, to see if they're really a problem. Also be sure to add substitutes for these foods. For example, if you eliminate milk, you may want to add calcium-fortified soya milk as a replacement. Here's a list of foods that are more likely to cause gas:

   - Asparagus
   - Beer
   - Broccoli
   - Brussels sprouts
   - Cabbage
   - Cauliflower
   - Cucumbers
   - Dried peas and beans
   - Fish
   - Melons
   - Milk
   - Nuts
   - Onion
   - Radishes
   - Soda
   - Yeast (and foods that encourage yeast production, such as sweets)

Since gas can result from incompletely digested foods, it may help to add foods to your diet that are known to improve digestion. For example, papaya and pineapple are both helpful, although raw pineapple shouldn't be taken if you're prone to blockages. Peppermint, fennel, and ginger teas are also useful for improving digestion and reducing gas.

How Do I Relieve Constipation With Diet?

When you're constipated, you either can't pass stool at all, or the stool that you do pass is small, dry, and passed with difficulty. This is a different problem from blockage: undigested food isn't blocking the stoma; instead, your digestive system is sluggish and having a hard time moving food through it as easily as it should. This problem affects those with colostomies almost exclusively. (Ileosotmy patients don't get constipated.) So, although reducing fiber intake often treats blockage, increasing it treats constipation. But be aware that in addition to increasing your fiber intake, you need to increase the amount of water you drink. Otherwise, your digestive system is going to have to deal with more stool without having anything to flush it through with.

If you have mild constipation, here are some tips to deal with it:

- Increase the amount of liquids you drink. Try to drink 8–10 glasses of water per day, in addition to any other liquids, such as milk and tea.
- Increase your intake of high fiber foods, such as bran and whole grain cereals, fresh fruit, raw and cooked vegetables, and whole grain breads. You may also want try a natural bulking agent, like psyllium seed, which can be found in a grocery or health food store. Remember to drink lots of water with it, or it'll make constipation even worse! Take one to two teaspoons of psyllium seed mixture twice daily with lots of water. Mix psyllium powder (found at many health food stores) with a cup of water and drink it. Follow with at least three cups of water.
- Add flax to your diet. Flax is a rich source of omega-3 fatty acids, and it's a proven stool softener and natural laxative. Take one to two tablespoons of flax seeds or flax seed oil per day. You can drizzle the uncooked oil on your cooked greens, or combine it with dried herbs and lemon juice to make a tasty salad dressing. Sprinkle the flax seeds on salads or bake them into nutritious muffins. Don't take flax if you're pregnant or breast-feeding, though, because some studies have shown it to have mild hormonal effects.
- Exercise daily. Even a twenty-minute walk is helpful.

How Do I Deal With Diarrhea?

There are a number of causes for diarrhea, or loose stools. Travel, contaminated water, and emotional distress can be factors. And if you have food poisoning, you're also likely to experience diarrhea. In these instances, both people with ileostomies and colostomies can experience diarrhea.

When none of these factors is the cause, then it's possible that something in your diet is causing problems for you. People with colostomies experience diarrhea as a result of diet less commonly than those with ileostomies. Experiment with this by removing a food from your diet, then adding it back a few weeks later and observing the effect. The following foods are common culprits:

- Baked beans
- Hot beverages
- Broccoli
- Chocolate
- Very large meals
- Heavily spiced foods
- Beer
- Soup
- Licorice
- Prune juice
- Dried beans
- Red wine

To deal with diarrhea, you need to eat foods that "bulk up" your stool. Foods like applesauce, pasta, bananas, boiled rice, and cheese can help this happen. Because it contains acidophilus, yogurt is also a good choice. Studies have found that acidophilus is useful in treating uncomplicated diarrhea, and taking acidophilus directly may yield more immediate results than eating yogurt. How much should you take? Acidophilus dosage is based on the number of live organisms in the acidophilus culture, and 1 to 10 billion viable organisms per day in divided doses is recommended. Acidophilus can be found in health food stores and some grocery stores. Natural bulking agents like psyllium, found in a grocery or health food store, also help firm up stool.

If you have diarrhea, it's also likely that you're losing lots of fluids. That's why it's especially critical to drink plenty of liquids, such as water, bouillon, and herbal tea. Ginger, fennel and peppermint teas, in particular, have a soothing effect on the digestive system.

If you have an ileostomy, it's especially important for you to replace the liquids, vitamins and minerals you're losing. If you don't, you run the risk of getting dehydrated and very ill.

If you're losing large amounts of fluid through your ileostomy because of diarrhea or other reasons (for example, you're playing sports in hot weather), you can drink a beverage like Gatorade to replace the lost fluids and minerals. Or you can make your own. One hospital's nutrition guide recommends the following recipe:

> 1 teaspoon of salt
> 4 teaspoons of corn syrup
> 1 teaspoon of baking soda
> 1 6-ounce can of frozen orange juice

Mix all ingredients together and add enough water to make one quart.

If dietary changes fail to improve the situation, your doctor may recommend medication to improve the diarrhea. This is usually quite successful.

If the diarrhea persists for more than 24 hours, or if you're feeling extremely ill, contact your doctor, in order to rule out infectious causes and in order to obtain proper treatment.

I Have an Ileostomy. How Do I Ensure that I Get Enough Minerals?

People who have ileostomies need to be mindful of the fact that potassium and sodium – two minerals required by the body to maintain health – are lost daily through the ileostomy. Before your ostomy surgery, the colon absorbed these minerals (as well as some water). Now that the colon has been removed, your body can't absorb these minerals as easily, and you run the risk of becoming depleted if you're not conscious of this.

Potassium and sodium loss can be remedied by including foods high in these minerals in your daily diet. Speak to your doctor if you have any health conditions that require that you limit your intake of either sodium or potassium (such as high blood pressure). In some cases, you may want to add mineral supplements to your diet, but consult your doctor before you do this. Normally, however, it's best to get sufficient amounts of these minerals from dietary sources. Here are some good dietary sources of potassium and sodium.

Foods high in potassium	Foods high in sodium
Dairy and carbohydrates: milk, potatoes. Meat: chicken, fish, pork, turkey, beef, duck, lamb, veal. Vegetables: lima beans, brussels sprouts, peppers, tomatoes, v8 juice, green beans, broccoli, spinach, tomato juice, avocado. Fruit and fruit juice: apricots, bananas, cherries, figs, grapefruit juice, nectarines, orange juice, peach nectar, plums, plum juice, prune juice, strawberries, apricot nectar, cantaloupe, dates, grapefruit, white grapes, oranges, peaches, pineapple, prunes, rhubarb,watermelon.	Condiments: ketchup, chili sauce, soy sauce, gravy, meat tenderizers, salts (celery, onion, garlic), Worcestershire sauce. Processed foods: canned and dried soups, sauces, canned meat, fish, stews and gravies, crackers and other snack foods, cold cuts, peanut butter, salad dressings, sausage, cheese, vegetables marinated or prepared in brine.

I Have a Urostomy. Do I Need to Make Changes to My Diet?

If you have a urostomy, you generally don't need to make changes to your diet to accommodate your ostomy. Unlike people with ileostomies, for example, you need not be concerned with reducing your intake of foods that may cause blockage, since your digestive system's function hasn't changed.

However, because you've had ostomy surgery, your body is going to need a well-balanced, nutritious diet to help it heal. So, this is a good opportunity for you to re-evaluate your diet and ensure that you're getting enough vitamins and minerals to support optimal health – and of course, to ensure that your diet is enjoyable! If possible, review your diet with a dietician to ensure that it supports your health in the best way possible.

It's also good to be aware of foods that can affect the color or odor of your urine. For example, beetroot can color urine red, and asparagus can give it a strong odor. Although discoloration and odor also happened before you got your ostomy, you may notice it now when you empty and change your pouch. Don't worry about discoloration; it's completely normal as long as you can trace it to foods that you ate.

As for odor, if the odor created by a certain food bothers you, you may want to eliminate it from your diet. Alternately, you can add a natural "internal deodorant," like parsley or chlorophyll, to your diet to neutralize the odor. Drinking lots of water also helps reduce odor, since it keeps the urine relatively clear. Drink 8–10 glasses per day unless your fluid intake is restricted. Keeping the urine acidic also helps reduce odor. You'll notice when your urine is alkaline because there may be a bluish discoloration of skin around the stoma. To acidify the urine, drink more water and other fluids – cranberry juice is especially helpful.

Skin Care

This section gives you basic information about how to take care of your ostomy and the skin around it. It also describes problems you might encounter with the skin around your ostomy, and tells you how to deal with them. Different skin problems can occur with different types of ostomies, and we'll look at the problems that are most likely for each.

But before we talk about what problems you may experience, it's probably a good idea to learn just what the skin around your stoma should look like. That way, you'll be in a position to judge whether you're having skin problems or not.

The skin surrounding your stoma should look much like the skin on the rest of your body. It should appear healthy and free of redness or discoloration. It's a good idea to check the skin of your stoma every time you change your pouch, so that you can notice any changes in the health of the skin early on and deal with them before they get painful.

Cleaning Your Stoma and the Skin around It

It's important to carefully clean your stoma and the skin around it. Since soap and water don't hurt the stoma, you can shower as you always have. Some people prefer to wear a pouch when they shower; this is fine too.

Although soap and water won't hurt the stoma, it isn't really necessary to use soap at all. If you do decide to use soap, choose one that's residue-free. Most moisturizing soaps, such as those that contain moisturizing cream, leave a filmy residue on the skin, even after rinsing. This can interfere with how well the adhesive adheres to your skin.

Although you'll need to use adhesives when changing your pouch, avoid letting the adhesive build up on your skin. This can irritate skin, causing redness and irritation. Remove adhesive with adhesive remover from an ostomy supplier. Remember to wipe this remover off your skin with water and then dry the skin around your stoma carefully before putting on a new pouch.

If you have a mucous fistula, take care of it the same way as you do your stoma. You may not need to clean it as frequently if there is little discharge. Between cleanings, cover it with a nonsterile, light dressing.

What Causes Skin Problems?

Pouches and other ostomy-related supplies such as adhesives and adhesive removers can be hard on the skin around the stoma. Skin can become irritated simply by pouch changes, so try to be gentle with your skin when you're changing your pouch, and dry your skin thoroughly before you put on a new pouch. Even so, this type of irritation is usually minimal if the skin is well cared for.

Skin problems can also be caused by the following:

Ill-fitting pouching systems

You'll know if your pouch isn't fitting correctly if the pouch contents leak onto the skin around the stoma, causing inflammation and redness. The pouch's opening may be too small or too big, or it may not fit your stoma if your stoma is irregularly shaped. The pouch fails to protect the skin around the stoma from contact with the stool or urine. When urine pools on the skin, the skin can look red, weepy, or waterlogged. And if stool touches the skin, the skin can become irritated and inflamed. The more caustic the stool, the more damage the stool can do. This tends to be a more common problem for people with ileostomies, since the stool is less formed and more caustic.

Sensitivity to ostomy products

If you constantly experience skin problems like redness, itchiness and irritation, it's possible that you're allergic to one of the products you use to take care of your stoma, such as the adhesive or skin barrier. If you have allergic reactions to a product, you may need to try different products to determine which works for you. Simply switching brands works for many people. If you're allergy-prone, it's best to "patch test" (try out) new products like adhesives or cement on another part of your body away from the stoma – the inside of the arm works well. That way, if you react to the product, it won't affect how well your appliance adheres to your body. If you're reacting to the material the pouch itself is made of, you may want to try covering the pouch with a soft, non-irritating pouch cover. You can make one yourself from any material, but commercial versions are also available.

Contact your ostomy supplier and ask if they have products for people with allergy-prone skin. You can also speak to your WOC nurse – he or she may know of products that are less likely to cause allergic reactions. Unfortunately for people with sensitive skin, it's mainly a trial and error process to find out what works and what doesn't.

Yeast infections

Yeast is a normal part of the digestive system, but it can become a problem if it multiplies and migrates to the skin around the stoma. This, combined with a moist environment within the pouch, can lead to a yeast infection. Signs of a yeast infection include red, itchy, inflamed skin.

Why do yeast infections occur? Some medications, such as antibiotics, can alter the balance of bacteria in your intestines, resulting in a yeast infection that extends to your skin. Or a yeast infection can occur as a result of a diet high in sugar and simple carbohydrates, combined with a moist environment within the pouch.

To deal with a yeast infection, try to keep the environment within the pouch as dry as possible, perhaps by using an ostomy protective powder or cream available from your ostomy supplier or doctor.

You may also want to try adding acidophilus supplements to your diet. Acidophilus helps counteract the overgrowth of yeast in your intestines by adding more good bacteria. Dosage is based on the number of live organisms in the acidophilus culture, and 1 to 10 billion viable organisms per day in divided doses is recommended. Acidophilus can be found in health food stores and some grocery stores. Remember to check the label to ensure that you're getting 1 to 10 billion live organisms.

Some herbal teas may also help treat yeast infections from the inside out. For example, Pau'arco tea is a well-known yeast fighter.

If none of these measures is working, you may also need to see your WOC nurse about using anti-fungal medications to re-balance the overgrowth of yeast in your body.

Hair under the pouch

Hair under the pouch can contribute to inflamed skin. To handle this, remove the hair around the stoma by trimming it with scissors or an electric razor. Always shave or trim with the blade pointing away from the stoma to avoid accidental injury. Don't use hair removal creams or lotions, since they can cause skin irritation.

Crystallized urine

If you have a urostomy, it's possible that urine may crystallize on the stoma, forming dry, irritating patches. To prevent this, each time you change your pouch, soak a washcloth in equal parts vinegar and water, then apply it to your stoma for a few minutes. Dry carefully before putting on your pouch.

Drinking lots of water also helps reduce crystallized urine by keeping the urine acidic. You may also want to add other sources of Vitamin C to your diet, or take Vitamin C supplements.

Medication

Normally, you don't have to change the way you take your medication after you get ostomy surgery. This is because most medications are absorbed in the small intestine. If you have a colostomy or urostomy, then your small intestine is completely intact and there's usually no change to the way these medications are absorbed. So you can take the same medications you did before, with little change.

If you have an ileostomy, things are a bit more complicated. You'll be happy to hear that most medications can be taken safely after ostomy surgery. The exceptions are "timed release" or "coated" medications. These may not be absorbed properly, since they're designed to be absorbed further down the digestive tract. As a result, they may be passed through your small intestine directly into the pouch, without being absorbed.

Here are some guidelines for dealing with medications when you have an ostomy.

- Inform your doctor and pharmacist that you have an ostomy, and review your medications with each of them. No matter what type of ostomy you have, it's best to review your medications with your doctor and WOC nurse to determine if you should make any changes. This includes all non-prescription medications (like vitamins and mineral supplements, aspirin, antacids, sugar and salt substitutes, anti-diarrhea medications, anti-inflammatory agents, and laxatives) as well as the birth control pill.

- Remind your doctor and pharmacist that you have an ostomy when new medications are prescribed for you. That way, you won't be prescribed a medication that isn't absorbed well by your body.

- When you have just started taking a new medication, check your pouch to see if it's been absorbed. If you notice that a pill has been passed into your pouch, contact your doctor or pharmacist to obtain an alternative medication.

- Do not crush or separate timed-release or enteric-coated tablets without checking with your doctor and pharmacist. If these medications are crushed, you may receive too much medication at once, which isn't good for your body.

- Keep a list of all the medications you're taking with you at all times – especially when you're traveling. You may also want to carry a medic alert card if your rectum has been removed. This card should state that you have an ostomy and that rectal enemas, suppositories, or rectal temperatures should not be attempted.

- Be aware that some medications, including vitamins and antibiotics, can change the way stool looks and smells. For example, regular use of pain medication can cause constipation. If you have a colostomy and are experiencing constipation (and you're taking pain medication regularly), see your doctor to determine if you can be treated with stool softeners or laxatives.

However, it's important to note that people with ileostomies generally shouldn't take stool softeners or laxatives. This is because ileostomy output is normally fairly loose, meaning that a fair amount of water and minerals are lost via the ileostomy. Loosening the stool further by using laxatives could lead to dehydration and electrolyte imbalance.

If you have a urostomy, you may notice that some medications change the color and odor of your urine. Antibiotics, vitamins, and pyridium are common culprits.

To reduce odor, drink lots of water (8-10 glasses per day unless your fluid intake is restricted). You may also want to try cranberry juice, which helps the urine stay acidic, thus reducing odor.

Some medications and supplements, such as Vitamin C, may help the urine stay acidic, but they can also cause urinary stones to form. If you take Vitamin C supplements, monitor your stoma carefully to ensure that there are no problems. In general, it's best to inform your doctor and pharmacist of all the medications (including vitamins) that you're taking, to avoid any problems down the road.

8

WORKING, PLAYING, AND SEEING THE WORLD

Taking Care of Business:
Dealing With Your Ostomy On the Job

Whether you're a member of a large corporation or work at home as a self-employed professional or homemaker, having an ostomy doesn't stop you from taking care of business.

During the recovery period following ostomy surgery, you should talk to your doctor about when you can return to work. Most people *can* return to the job they were doing before surgery. There are a few exceptions, though. Jobs that require heavy lifting or are performed in a very hot environment may require that you take extra precautions. For example, if you need to lift very heavy objects, you may want to wear sturdy support garments to decrease strain on your abdominal area. And if your work environment is so hot that you sweat a lot, ensure that you drink extra fluids to make up for those lost. Speak to your doctor about your options.

You may want to ask your employer if you can work from home or part-time for the first few weeks you're back at work. This lets you take rest breaks when you need to, since your body may still be tired from surgery. It also lets you get accustomed to dealing with an ostomy in the workplace in a gradual way, especially if you're worried about "accidents" occurring as you gain experience with caring for your ostomy. Also, since ostomies tend to be more temperamental at the beginning, the freedom to take frequent breaks to "check in" with your ostomy can be helpful. In reality, accidents are rare, but many people find that keeping extra appliances and a change of clothing at work helps them feel more secure.

Keep in mind that you don't have to tell everyone at work about your ostomy. It's likely that because you had to take time off for surgery, your immediate supervisor or manager knows about it. But even they need not know that you now have an ostomy, if you feel more comfortable that way. They only need to know that you had surgery, and that you're healthy now. One reason you want to share this information with them is that you may want access to private toilet facilities, if they're available. But again, the choice is yours.

Many people choose not to tell any of their peers, or they may tell a few trusted friends. Others like to share more readily. The key is to do what's comfortable for you.

Ostomies and the Sporting Life

One thing is for sure: if you're a confirmed couch potato, you can't use your ostomy as an excuse!

If you have an ostomy, you can swim, ski, snowboard, go inline skating, bike, hike, ride horses, play baseball, learn Tai Chi and even run marathons. In short, you can do any sport or activity that interests you (although you need to take care to protect the stoma when playing heavy contract sports like football, hockey, karate and wrestling).

The key is to start gradually and build up your level of activity as you see fit. Rome wasn't built in a day, and you're unlikely to become an Olympian in a hurry, either. You need to start slowly and listen to your body as you go – especially if you weren't active before you had an ostomy (and if you had IBD, it's likely that your illness didn't allow you to be).

To start, it's a good idea to work out an exercise and diet plan with your doctor, so that you can be sure you're getting enough nutrients and you're not overdoing it. This is especially important if you have an ileostomy, since vigorous activity in hot weather can deplete your body of fluids and minerals very quickly. That's because you no longer have a colon and the colon was responsible for absorbing water and minerals. Drink lots of water and electrolyte-rich drinks like Gatorade during strenuous exercise or hot weather, and you should do fine.

Here are some more tips to help you plan an exercise regimen that suits you.

- Swimming is a good exercise to start with. It's non-impact – making it gentle on the body – and it provides an excellent cardiovascular workout.

- Walking and hiking are good ways to keep fit. Early in your recovery, you may want to limit yourself to short, easy walks. But as you progress, you can challenge yourself with more strenuous hikes – and enjoy fresh air and nature to boot!
- Yoga is a gentle way to awaken the body after a long period of inactivity. It can also be a good way to maintain a healthy body and mind over the long term. Be careful with any postures that involve abdominal muscles, such as forward and backward bends, since yours have been through a workout already due to surgery and may take awhile to get back into form. It's best to start with a restorative yoga class taught by a certified yoga instructor. Check with your local yoga studio for more information.

In fact, being active has many benefits for your mind, as well as your body. As Michael, 35, remarks:

Back before I got my ileostomy, I couldn't really participate in sports at all. I was too busy running to the bathroom most of the time, and going hiking or swimming was out of the question. After surgery, I wasn't in constant pain anymore, but I was still worried about taking part in sports. I worried that my pouch would leak, and that I would hurt the stoma and end up sick all over again. Instead of throwing myself right into heavy-duty sports, I decided to start slowly. First I tried swimming, and I had to take a few precautions like using waterproof tape around my pouch. I also wore a belt with a flap that goes over the pouch – that made me feel more secure that the pouch wouldn't come off while I was in the water. Since then, I've enjoyed all sorts of activities, from snowboarding to competitive cycling. Being able to be so active has made me feel better about my ostomy, since I couldn't have done many of the things I'm doing now when I was sick.

On the Road with an Ostomy

When you found out that you were getting an ostomy, you may have wondered if you would ever travel again. Well, take heart. Traveling is not only an option with an ostomy, but many people who had ostomy surgery as a result of IBD will find it less stressful than it was before. No more memorizing the locations of all the restrooms in every city on your itinerary, and no more hoping desperately that your colitis won't flare up while you're staying at your fastidious Aunt Hilda's. You may have felt at the mercy of your IBD – as though anything could happen, at any time. Thanks to your ostomy, this kind of anxiety-creating situation isn't going to be an issue anymore. Now the control of your digestive and urinary systems is back in your hands.

The key to traveling well with an ostomy is good planning, coupled with an awareness of all the resources available to you. The following guidelines will help you plan a trip free of anxiety, whether it be for business or pleasure.

Get travel insurance

Get travel insurance for the country that you're visiting. That way, if something happens, you won't need to worry about astronomical expenses.

Bring a written summary of your surgical and medical history

When you travel, bring a written summary of your medical and surgical history (actually, this is useful to keep on hand whether you plan to travel or not). Include current medications, allergies to foods or medications, and physicians' names, addresses and telephone numbers. If a relative or friend has power of attorney or is a health proxy, or if there is a living will, note this as well. You may also choose to include copies of operative notes and discharge summaries from recent or complex procedures and hospitalizations. If you wish, obtain a copy of your full medical record, and take that with you, too. You may also want to wear a Medic-Alert bracelet to ensure that any caregivers treating you at your destination are aware that you have an ostomy

If your trip is longer than one week, you may also want to notify your doctor of your travel plans and ask for the name and number of a physician at your destination.

Compile a list of contacts at your destination

In addition to getting the name of a physician at your destination, you may also want to bring along the hotline number for ostomy suppliers and ostomy organizations at your destination as well. For example, the United Ostomy Association can provide you with a list of ostomy groups pertinent to your trip. And some ostomy suppliers, such as Convatec, offer a help line number that you can call while traveling, in case you run into problems with your appliance. See the Resources section for more information.

Plan your route

If you're traveling by car, plan a road route that includes frequent comfort stops. If possible, the stops should have "disabled" toilets, making it easier for you to empty and change pouches and wash appliances.

Bring extra supplies

Bring about double the amount of supplies you'd normally use in the timeframe of your trip. This allows for possible travel delays, as well as bowel upsets resulting from foreign food and water intake.

Put together a travel set of ostomy supplies

Some ostomy suppliers sell special travel supplies that include items especially useful for traveling, such as several travel kits with special pockets, a hook, a mirror, and scissors. Because airport security can be stringent, you may want to get a doctor's note stating that you need these supplies as a result of a medical condition.

It's also helpful to add the following items to your travel set:

- plastic bags with twist ties for soiled tissues and appliances;
- pre-moistened towelettes for cleaning hands (these are available from most grocery and drug stores);
- a folding plastic cup for rinsing appliances, just in case the facilities aren't up to par;
- an extra appliance with a pre-sized opening; and
- toilet tissue – again, just in case it's not available at your destination.

Keep your supplies with you

Always keep your ostomy supplies in your hand luggage. Some airlines allow you to bring extra hand luggage on board for medical supplies; check with your airline when you're booking your flight.

Keep supplies at a moderate temperature

If you're traveling in a hot climate, keep your appliances as cool as possible to avoid the potential melting of adhesives. A cool, shady place is best, but don't put them in the refrigerator. Conversely, if you're traveling in a cold climate, keep the supplies inside the car rather than in the trunk.

Eat regularly

To minimize the impact of travel on your body, eat regularly and as close to your normal diet as possible. If you have special dietary requirements, ask the airline if special meals are available when you're booking your flight. Avoid carbonated drinks and alcohol on airplanes; these exacerbate the dehydrating impact of air pressure changes during the flight.

Watch your food and water intake

Be careful with your intake of food and water. Although you should drink lots of water, especially if it's hot, try and make it bottled (with seal intact) instead of the local tap variety. Avoid ice cubes and salads. Eat fruit in moderation to avoid diarrhea. Take anti-diarrhea medication with you, if you have it.

If you irrigate, use bottled water to irrigate as well.

Book an aisle seat

Booking an aisle seat may relieve stiffness and pain that can result from ostomy surgery by allowing you to frequently change body position and stretch your legs.

Book a seat near the toilet

Sitting near the toilets will allow you quick and easy access to them if needed, and will help you avoid the inevitable line-ups.

Wear a seat belt

If you're traveling by car, always wear a seat belt. If fitted properly, the seat belt shouldn't interfere with your ostomy. If your seat belt is uncomfortable, try putting a piece of foam under the belt and over your appliance.

Take it easy on the beach

Yes, you should enjoy yourself by lazing on the beach, but try to spend only moderate amounts of time in the sun at first. Remember to drink lots of fluids – preferably bottled water with the seal intact – and, if you have an ileostomy, make sure that you're not losing too much salt in your sweat. Keep lots of water and electrolyte-rich drinks like Gatorade on hand so that you can replace lost fluids and minerals.

As for swimming – you can swim in either sea or pool, but you must wear a pouch at all times. It's also best to wear waterproof tape around your appliance. Women can wear one-piece suits, and if the location of the stoma is convenient, bikinis as well. Men are often better off with boxer-style swimsuits but, again, whatever you're comfortable with works best for you. Men may also want to wear a gentle support belt to keep the appliance in place under the bathing suit. If you have trouble finding a swimsuit that works with your ostomy, there are special swimsuit stores that offer suits especially designed for people with ostomies. See the Resources section at the end of this book for more information.

Travel Tips for Irrigation

Make sure your irrigation water is pure

In general, if the water isn't safe to drink, it's not safe for irrigation either. If you're in doubt about the purity of the water for irrigating, you can try one of the following:

- Add two tablets of halazone (a water purifier) per quart of water. Because halazone dissolves slowly, it's best to add it to hot water and then let the water cool before using.
- Use a portable water purifier. See the Resources section for more information.
- Add a two percent tincture of iodine to the irrigation water. For one quart of water, add five drops if the water is clear; ten drops if it's cloudy, then let stand for thirty minutes before using.
- Use soda water – but make sure you let it go flat first!

Carry a plastic sheet and a bent coat hanger

The plastic sheet can be put on the floor to protect it from spillage, and the coat hanger can be placed over the shower rod. You can then hang the enema bag on it.

Irrigate at night rather than in the morning

If you're traveling in the morning, it's best to irrigate at night to avoid rushing and a potentially unproductive irrigation.

Carry extra appliances

Because traveling may upset your normal bowel patterns, it's best to carry a supply of appliances just in case irrigation isn't successful for you – or if you experience bowel upset or diarrhea.

For more travel tips

The United Ostomy Association offers a number of excellent publications that will provide you with information about traveling with an ostomy. See the Resources section of this book, and check with your local chapter for more information.

9
BODY IMAGE, RELATIONSHIPS AND SEXUALITY

> I kept thinking how lucky I was that I was already married, because it would be even more horrendous trying to date with an ileostomy.
> —*From a woman with an ileostomy*

> Throughout my illness, the thought that it would destroy my marriage, and make my wife feel she was married to "damaged goods," bothered me. But my wife has told me that she married me for who I am, for my heart. To her, I'm exactly the same as I was before surgery.
> —*From a man with an ileostomy*

Do these comments sound familiar? Do they echo the thoughts you have or have had about your ostomy and its impact on you? It's not surprising if they do. The presence of a stoma, and the physical reality that your body and its functioning has been changed, inevitably change the way you relate to yourself. It can change the way you relate to others as well. But after an initial adjustment period, it can mean greater self-confidence in the long run. That's because successfully handling challenges leads to increased self-reliance – and since an ostomy is one heck of a challenge, you can expect to become one heck of a self-assured person once you've learned to manage it!

Having an ostomy not only changes your physical body and how you perceive it, but it can also mean changes to the way you function sexually. Obviously this can present difficulties for both women and men.

Directly following ostomy surgery, you'll likely be more concerned about survival than sex. Ostomy surgery, and the bowel and bladder disease that preceded it, are serious matters. Most people experience some level of apprehension both before and after surgery. Some people who have surgery for cancer may worry that the cancer isn't gone, or that it's spread.

Usually, however, after survival is assured, people with new ostomies begin to make adjustments to their new body image, and become familiar with their body's changes. That's often around the time when the question of sexuality comes up. You may begin to wonder how having an ostomy will affect your sex life. Will it prevent you from enjoying sex? Will it make you undesirable to potential partners? The answer is that having an ostomy usually doesn't mean any changes in sexual function for women or men. Both may experience some changes, with the situation being somewhat more complex for men. But the good news is that problems are usually temporary. Even if a problem proves permanent, there are solutions – as a good many men and women happy with themselves and their sex lives can attest!

You Have the Right to Sexual Health

Remember that you have the right to full sexual health, and to any information or treatments that can help you achieve it. Some studies have shown that people with new ostomies sometimes feel guilty about wanting a full sex life. They may feel that they should be grateful for the life-saving surgery, and have no right to expect sexual fulfillment on top of that.

If that's true for you, then realize that the physical, sexual and emotional health aspects of total health are intimately linked. There's no doubt about it – an ostomy improves your physical vitality. But if physical improvement isn't accompanied by a heightened enjoyment of life – which includes sex and romantic relationships – then it's just not as valuable as it could be.

All people, with or without ostomies, have the right to sexual health. To enjoy full sexual health, the World Health Organization (WHO) has identified that a person must have:

- The capacity to enjoy and control sexual and reproductive behavior in accordance with social and personal ethics.

- Freedom from fear, shame, guilt, misconceptions and other psychological factors that inhibit the sexual response and impair sexual relationships.
- Freedom from organic disorders, disease and deficiencies that may interfere with either sexual or reproductive function or both.

Too often when it comes to sex, people with new ostomies don't get the information and support they need from their healthcare providers. Doctors and nurses may not be comfortable enough with the subject matter to raise the topic of sexuality, and the person with a new ostomy usually has enough to think about without having to worry about broaching a potentially difficult subject.

It's important to find a professional who's comfortable discussing issues about your sexuality with you. If you're finding that your healthcare provider is unable or unwilling to discuss these issues, or if you have specific concerns that you feel can't be addressed adequately by him or her, you may need to ask for referrals to another doctor, WOC nurse or specialist.

For example, you may prefer to work with a urologist or sex therapist who specializes in physical and psychological sexual issues. Or, if you're gay or lesbian, you may prefer to work with healthcare professionals familiar with gay sexuality. In any case, don't hesitate to get the support you need. You deserve it.

The Grieving Process

Whether you have a conventional or a continent ostomy, your perception of your body has been altered considerably. Our society has many taboos about the elimination organs and waste products. Most people would just as soon forget about how their body eliminates waste, and here you are with a constant reminder. The adjustments to this new way of being are considerable. They make great demands on you: you need to be patient, flexible, and have a sense of humor.

Because you're experiencing changes to your body image, you're probably also experiencing some of the difficult emotions that go along with them. Feelings of sadness and even depression, angry outbursts, and irritability are all signs that you're making the emotional adjustments necessary to live well with your ostomy. It may not seem like it at the time, but these emotions will eventually lead to self-acceptance. It's actually less perilous to acknowledge and express these perfectly normal emotions than it is to repress them. During any crisis, denial is a healthy reaction – it protects you from harsh realities that you may not be ready to accept yet. But remaining in a state of denial and putting your life on hold won't benefit you in the long run.

It may help for you to remember that what's happening to you is a grieving process. You've lost part of yourself, and you're experiencing grief over the loss. It's quite okay – and in fact it's normal – for you to experience negative emotions about yourself and your ostomy. The key is to observe them, confront them, and eventually overcome them. Time helps, and so does an understanding of the five stages of the grieving process.

1. In the first stage, "realization," you may experience avoidance or denial of your loss. You may feel distanced from the world, as if what's happened to you isn't real.

2. Fear and anxiety characterize the next stage, which is called "alarm." You've realized that you now have an ostomy, and are beginning to understand what it means to live with one. You may not have developed the practical or emotional coping skills required to deal with this reality, which leads to anxiety and fear.

3. This stage leads into a sense of "searching," in which you may be preoccupied with your loss and experience intense feelings of anger, anxiety or even panic.

4. Then, in the "grief" stage, you begin to really acknowledge your loss. You may feel mutilated or violated, and experience intense feelings of sadness and loss.

5. With time and the right support, the "resolution" stage arrives. You have learned to cope with your ostomy in both practical and emotional terms, and have successfully adjusted your sense of yourself as able to deal with your new reality. You may experience this stage as a feeling of internal calm, or peace. Knowing that you've overcome such a tough obstacle can leave you with a sense of accomplishment and a greater appreciation of yourself.

There are no hard and fast rules about how long each stage of grief will last. That's because you're unique and you'll grieve at your own pace and in your own way. Keep in mind, too, that you're unlikely to make your way through the stages in an orderly way. You may feel fine one day, but the next day find that you're angry and depressed again. That's normal, and it's important to treat yourself with as much gentleness and patience as you'd treat a loved one if they were in your shoes.

But if you find that the grieving process is so long-lasting that it interferes with your personal and professional relationships and with your ability to carry on your day-to-day activities, you may want to consider counseling. Short-term counseling can be very helpful in allowing you to overcome the "humps" on your way to emotional healing.

It can also be useful to know that other people have gone through what you're going through, and not only have they survived, but – more importantly – they thrived. The United Ostomy Association has a visiting program that can be very helpful in this capacity. It matches you up with people who've successfully adjusted to the new self-image that ostomy surgery brings. They'll visit you as many (or as few) times as you need them to. Their support can be of great help to you.

Keep in mind, too, that your partner may be experiencing some or all of these emotions as well. Counseling, either singly or as a couple, is always a good option if these emotions become overwhelming or don't seem to be fading in intensity over time.

His and Hers: How Will Your Ostomy Affect Your Sex Life?

Most people – both female and male – who get ostomy surgery are worried about how the ostomy will affect their sex life. They may worry that it may physically interfere with sex, or, worse, make them less desirable to their partners.

These fears are understandable, and need to be addressed. But the reality is that, given an adjustment period, your ostomy is unlikely to affect your ability to satisfy yourself and your partner sexually. It may take time, some creativity and even a sense of humor for those times the ostomy decides to "speak up" during lovemaking – but these are challenges that are quite possible to overcome.

There are several ways your ability to be sexual may be affected by ostomy surgery.

On a physical level, sometimes ostomy surgery can damage the nerve endings in the genital area. It's also more likely to cause sexual problems for those who've had colostomies or urostomies due to cancer than for those who've had ileostomies due to IBD. That's because the surgical technique for cancer surgeries can sometimes damage the pelvic nerves and blood supply to the genitals. One sobering study reported that 70–80 percent of men with colostomies report sexual problems. Sexual problems for women were lower, ranging from five to 30 percent. Full recovery of sexual functioning is often achieved, though it may take months (or in rare cases, years) for the nerves to regain sufficient blood supply to react as they once did to sexual stimulation.

Before worrying about nerve damage, though, remember that a lack of sexual desire is common in the months following ostomy surgery. Both body and mind are occupied with the vital job of healing, which will probably make you feel fatigued. Most people who undergo major surgery experience this, whether or not the surgery resulted in an ostomy. It's important to give your body a rest – and yourself a break.

On a brighter note, some studies indicate that both males and females with new ileostomies report unchanged or improved sexual relationships – perhaps because IBD made sex so difficult before surgery.

How Soon Can I Have Sex After Surgery?

So how soon after your surgery can you engage in sex? That depends on what you think of as sex. Many of us have a narrow definition of what it means to be sexual, limiting ourselves to intercourse as the "main course," with perhaps a bit of foreplay as an appetizer.

Unfortunately, this limited concept of sex often leads to anxiety in the bedroom. If we can't "perform" sexually by getting an erection or having an orgasm, then suddenly we become "impotent" or "frigid."

These two words – impotent and frigid – represent the rather limited, restrictive concept of sex that's common. Most of us – with or without an ostomy – would benefit by looking at sexuality from a more open standpoint. The brain has been called the most important sex organ in the body – use it to think of creative ways to satisfy your partner sexually. And the skin has been called the largest sex organ in the body – a fact to which lovers who enjoy sensual massage can attest. There are many good sex manuals available at your local library or bookstore. All can help enhance your sexual creativity.

That said, it's usually best to refrain from intercourse until you're both physically and emotionally sufficiently recovered from your surgery. That doesn't mean you should be 100 percent recovered – just that you've regained enough energy and vitality to become interested in sex again. Don't force yourself. There's nothing less sexually appealing than experiencing pain from your healing incisions during sexplay.

Abdominal surgery is very taxing on the body, and limits all types of vigorous activity – including sexual activity. The amount of time you need to wait will depend on how you feel, and on your doctor's advice. It's different for different people; for example, it might depend on how ill you were prior to surgery, or on how comfortable you feel with your new ostomy and your altered body image. And be aware that your first amorous encounters after ostomy surgery may not be what you'd like them to be. Have patience with yourself, and things just might pick up from there.

Kiss and Tell: When Should You Tell a New Partner About Your Ostomy?

It can be a bonding experience when you and your partner gradually become accustomed to your ostomy together. But when should you tell a new partner about your ostomy? The answer isn't the same for everyone. Some people are happy adhering to the common advice: tell when discovery is imminent. Others are more comfortable divulging the information before this, because they feel much closer to the other person once "the cat is out of the bag." Sharing about something as intimate as an ostomy often leads to a deeper trust between partners, and trust typically makes sex that much more satisfying when it does occur. Imagine telling your partner and receiving a warm, supportive response – isn't that more likely to make you feel closer to him or her? And if the supportive response isn't forthcoming immediately, give the person the benefit of the doubt. It took you awhile to adjust to your ostomy, and it's likely to take your partner some time too.

Even the worst case scenario – flat-out rejection, blamed on the ostomy – is probably not really about the ostomy at all. And if someone rejects you for having an ostomy, is that person really a worthy recipient of your interest in the first place?

So when should you tell? There's no hard and fast rule, although it's only respectful of the other person to inform them before they find out for themselves – or before you get married, whichever is first!

It's often helpful to remember that most people have fears and doubts about their bodies, and some have information that they, like you, need to divulge before intimacy occurs. So you're not alone in worrying about whether to kiss first and tell later, or the other way around.

How should you tell your partner? A simple, straightforward explanation is best. Your partner may have lots of questions. Answer them simply, without going into excessive detail or making apologies. How comfortable you are with your ostomy will show clearly in this conversation. The more self-accepting you are, the more likely your partner will be to accept you as well.

Women and Their Ostomies

How will my sex life change?

On the physical level, women usually experience little change to their *physical* sexual functioning, defined as the ability to experience sexual pleasure and orgasm. That's because the surgical site for the creation of an ostomy is farther away from a woman's sex organs than it is from a man's.

You're most likely to experience problems if you had your rectum removed as part of ostomy surgery. Removal of the rectum can affect pelvic blood flow and nerve supply to the vagina, vulva and uterus, which in turn can affect your ability to become sexually aroused and experience orgasm. As well, it's possible that the scarring that occurred at the surgical site could result in a narrowing of the vagina. You'd experience this during sexual activity as loss of sensation, discomfort, vaginal dryness and even dyspareunia (pain during intercourse).

Luckily, these symptoms tend to decrease in severity and even disappear entirely in the years following surgery. One study indicates that 77 percent of women experience some level of pain during intercourse in the first year following their surgery, but that the symptoms decrease over time.

If you're taking medication for pain, or are undergoing chemotherapy or radiation treatment for cancer, then keep in mind that these can affect your sexual function as well.

This doesn't mean that you have to live with painful or uncomfortable sex – or live without sex altogether. If you're experiencing any of these symptoms, consult your doctor. He or she should be able to offer you concrete suggestions to alleviate these symptoms and make sex what it should be – a satisfying and pleasurable experience. For example, women experiencing vaginal dryness may want to try one of the many good lubricants available to help this problem. Replens and KY-Jelly are just two. Ask your doctor or gynecologist for more recommendations on how to make sex more comfortable.

You may also experience a lack of sexual desire after ostomy surgery. Keep in mind that this is normal – it's common to experience a temporary decrease in sexual desire and sexual activity following any major surgery. Most women find that their interest in sex reverts back to previous levels if they give themselves time to adjust to the new ostomy.

For the small number of women who get ostomies as part of extensive pelvic surgery for cancer, the challenges will be greater – both on a physical and emotional level. This surgery can involve the removal of the uterus, bowel, bladder and genitals, leading to obvious challenges to sexual functioning. Although this surgery usually represents the only chance for long-term survival, it can be devastating to a woman's ability to experience sexual pleasure, and her ability to feel good about her body. Some women choose to have a re-constructed vagina created as part of their surgery, which can increase feelings of sexual attractiveness. But the ability to experience sexual pleasure will be diminished or gone.

However, this situation is rare. Most women who get ostomies as the result of IBD or colon cancer can count on a full, if gradual, return to their previous enjoyment of sex.

Body Image

Although the physical problems you may experience after surgery can be difficult, probably the biggest hurdle that you have to face after ostomy surgery isn't your physical recovery – it's your emotional recovery.

If you're experiencing problems with feeling sexually attractive after ostomy surgery, you're not alone. Having an ostomy is a change to the way you feel about your body, and you may be worried that your partner (or any potential partner) won't be attracted to you now that you have an ostomy.

Ostomy surgery means a major shift in your body image. Body image is the way you see yourself – the attitude you have toward your body. Most women need to take their time in adapting to these changes. Some may even choose to get counseling, if the problems persist and interfere with their quality of life. It's not unusual, for example, to experience a resurgence of issues about how you feel about yourself and your sexuality. These issues may have existed before, but now they seem more concrete. It's as if the ostomy becomes a way to externalize them.

After getting her ileostomy, 23-year-old Melanie felt nervous whenever she met an attractive, eligible man. If he showed interest, she was initially excited and responsive. But then fear of her ileostomy being discovered seemed to catch hold of her, and she began to back away. This pattern continued for two years after her surgery, causing Melanie great anguish. She felt frustrated that she couldn't maintain a relationship, even though she knew she wanted one. This compounded her feelings of self-blame – not only was she scared of someone finding out about her ostomy, she blamed herself for her fear! During counseling, Melanie was able to confront that her fear of self-exposure pre-dated her ostomy surgery. In fact, her ostomy was only one of the things about herself that made her feel vulnerable – and perhaps the least threatening at that. She discovered that she'd projected all her doubts about herself onto her ostomy, and used it to protect herself emotionally. Once she realized this, her self-image improved and she gained self-confidence – something that's often the most attractive attribute of all!

But sometimes the emotions connected to your ostomy are about physical issues as well as psychological ones. If you had surgery due to cancer, for example, you may be worried that the cancer isn't gone, or that it's spread. Discuss these fears with your WOC nurse and doctor. Many women find getting clear, complete and accurate information about the risk factors is helpful to maintaining peace of mind.

Many women would benefit from an increase in awareness about their sexuality; this is where a good sex manual is helpful. Lonnie Barbach's classic, *For Yourself: The Fulfillment of Female Sexuality* is a good one. Check the Resources section for more suggestions.

What About Pregnancy?

You'll be happy to hear that pregnancy is not only possible when you have an ostomy, but some women find that there are actually advantages to having a baby when you have an ostomy. Hemorrhoids, for example, are not likely to occur if you've had an abdominoperineal resection. And if you have an ileostomy, you're certainly not going to get constipated!

With good prenatal care, there's no reason your pregnancy should differ from any other woman's. However, there are a few things to consider before getting pregnant, while you're carrying the baby, during delivery, and after delivery.

Before the Baby

It's best to wait at least a year after ostomy surgery before getting pregnant. This allows the body to heal sufficiently from the surgery, and lets you adjust to your new body image before changing it again through pregnancy.

If you had IBD for years prior to surgery, it may be best to wait even longer, so that the body can replenish its depleted stores of vitamins and minerals. Two years is the recommended amount of time to wait in this case.

During Your Pregnancy

As your belly begins to expand, you may experience some annoying but relatively minor problems with your appliances.

First and most annoyingly, you may have problems seeing and changing your pouch as your belly grows. Experiment with different pouching systems to find the one that's easiest for you to manage. You may find a one-piece pouching system works better than a two-piece one. One-piece systems may be easier for you to manage because they're often softer and more flexible.

The stoma position and shape may change, too, as your abdominal contour changes. This is normal, and will likely return to normal after delivery.

Due to changes in hormone balance, you may find that your pouch becomes "stickier" than it was before, making it more difficult to remove than you're used to.

Conversely, and for the same reason, your appliance may not adhere as well as it did before. As a result, you may need to experiment a bit with your adhesives to find one that works for you.

If you notice that your stoma is retracting into your abdomen as your belly expands, don't worry. This is normal. It may help for you to use a convex appliance to prevent leakage, since stomas that are more retracted tend to be harder to fit properly with an appliance. Be sure to check with your WOC nurse if you decide to switch to a convex appliance. If used inappropriately, they can be damaging to the stoma.

As with all other pregnant women, it's important for you to ensure that you get plenty of fluids (especially if you have an ileostomy) and watch your diet. If you have a colostomy and experience constipation, review your diet and fluid intake first. See your doctor if the problem persists – it's best not to self-treat by taking laxatives.

If you have a urostomy, you'll need to take extra care to avoid urinary tract infections. Check with your doctor for preventative measures. Cranberry juice is an easy and healthy way to both prevent and treat urinary tract infections. Have a glass a day of pure, unsweetened juice (you may want to sweeten it with honey or another sweetener, since pure cranberry juice is quite bitter).

If you had ostomy surgery because of familial polyposis, be aware that your children will be at risk for the disease as well and, like you, may require bowel surgery. Consult your doctor for more information.

Are there problems that might occur because of the proximity of the baby and your stoma? Well, it's possible, though unlikely, that some pregnancies may apply pressure to the surgical site, which can cause cramps and pain. Make sure that your doctor and the hospital staff are aware of your surgical history, so that they don't mistake these cramps for labor pains.

During and After Delivery

For women with ostomies, as for most other women, vaginal delivery is the norm. If your surgery included an abdominoperineal resection, be sure to inform your doctor of this well before your due date. In fact, it's best for the staff of the hospital to be familiar with ostomy care, and with the changed internal structure of your abdomen.

You could suggest that your obstetrician speak with your surgeon, so that he or she fully understands the organization of your GI or urinary tract. This is especially important if you've had ileoanal pouch surgery. That's because if a Cesarean section is necessary, the operating surgeon should be fully aware of the pouch beforehand. Of course, a Cesarean section is unlikely to be required, and it has nothing to do with having an ostomy. However, it's always best to be prepared.

After the birth, most people notice that their stomas return to their pre-pregnancy size and shape. Some women report that they're actually happier with their post-natal stoma: if the stoma was retracted prior to surgery (and therefore harder to manage), it may protrude more readily from the abdomen, making it easier to manage than it was before.

What If I Don't Want to Have a Baby?

Contraception is as important an issue for women with ostomies as it is for those without. Generally speaking, you have the same contraceptive choices as do women without ostomies. Unlike women without ostomies, however, you need to consider how your chosen method of birth control works with your altered gastrointestinal tract.

For example, if you dealt with years of IBD, your periods may have stopped. This is because your body wasn't getting enough nutrients to produce a monthly period. Once your nutritional reservoirs are replenished, however, you'll likely become fertile again within a few months. It's important for you to take precautions, and be aware of the limitations of the different methods of birth control.

Having an ostomy can affect how well the contraceptive pill works for you. Low-dose contraceptives, for example, are often not adequately absorbed in women who have an ileostomy or a colostomy, and the protection they offer from pregnancy is significantly reduced.

Most medications, such as those for IBD, won't interfere with the effectiveness of the contraceptive pill. Keep in mind, however, that there's some evidence that the use of the oral contraceptive pill may trigger acute flare-ups of Crohn's disease.

Discuss the options with your doctor to determine the best method of birth control for you.

Men and Their Ostomies

The majority of men enjoy the same level of sexual pleasure as before ostomy surgery. Some enjoy sex even more than they did before – especially if the surgery was done as a result of years of suffering from IBD. In fact, one study indicates that 12 percent of men with new ileostomies actually experience an increase in frequency of sexual intercourse after surgery!

Of course, you need to give yourself enough time to recover from the surgery. It's unlikely that you're going to be able to hop into bed with your partner a week after surgery and have hours of uninterrupted sex!

Some men, however, do experience physical changes in how they function sexually after ostomy surgery. Luckily, most are temporary for most men, although you may have to have patience with yourself and explore your options.

Sexual difficulties are more likely if you had colostomy surgery with an abdominoperineal resection as a result of colon or rectal cancer, or if you had urostomy surgery for bladder cancer. That's because lower bowel and bladder surgery involves the removal of some organs in the pelvic area. This can damage nerves and impede blood supply to the genitals. It can also result in direct scarring.

Problems vary, depending on the extent of nerve damage, and fortunately they're usually temporary. Issues include a decrease in sexual activity and reduced sex drive, as well as the following:

- Difficulty having or maintaining an erection (erectile dysfunction). Also known as impotence, this is a failure to get an erection, or a failure to maintain an erection for satisfactory intercourse.
- Retrograde ejaculation with "dry orgasm." Retrograde ejaculation happens when semen travels to the bladder rather than out the urethra (the tube running from the bladder through the penis to the outside). You'll still have an erection and orgasm, but no ejaculate, or semen, will be visible. Why does retrograde ejaculation occur? For ejaculation to occur normally, the opening of the bladder into the urethra must close so that the semen doesn't enter it. If the opening doesn't close properly, retrograde ejaculation occurs. Since ejaculation is controlled by nerves to the bladder, if they're damaged (as they could be by ostomy surgery), control of this opening is lost and retrograde ejaculation occurs.

Treatments for these conditions are available. Since it's the most common problem after ostomy surgery, treatment options for erectile dysfunction are outlined below. As you're exploring your options, it's important that you speak to your doctor to find out which ones are appropriate for you.

Treating Erectile Dysfunction

Before you make any decisions about treatment options to restore erectile functioning, it's important to learn as much as you can about the available choices, so you can make an informed decision and choose the option that works best for you.

Also, if you have a partner or a spouse, involve them in the decision making process. Whatever method you choose should be compatible with the way you and your partner enjoy sex.

If you have difficulty talking about your sexual needs and preferences with your partner, counseling may be helpful. With efforts made in this area, you may end up with the "side benefit" of a more open and communicative relationship with your partner.

Here are some options for treating erectile difficulties.

Penile Implants

Contrary to popular belief, you don't need to ejaculate or have an erection to enjoy sexual sensation and orgasm. Erections occur due to increased blood flow into the penis. When nerves are damaged, increased blood flow no longer takes place, and a normal erection isn't possible. Since the increased blood flow necessary to achieve normal erection is no longer possible, a penile implant can give an erection rigid enough for sexual intercourse. The implant doesn't replace the sensation of a normal erection, but you'll still experience orgasm and ejaculation because they occur independently of erection.

Complications can include mechanical failure of the device and infection (about 10 percent of men have complications). The cost is usually covered by insurance when a medical problem has been documented, but Medicare and some insurance companies may not cover the entire cost.

Penile implants are available in two basic types: semi-rigid malleable rods and hydraulic inflatables. The former keep the penis in a permanent semi-rigid state. They're popular because they're relatively easy to implant, have a low mechanical failure rate, and are simple to operate. They're also cheaper than the hydraulic inflatable penile implants. However, some men find a permanently rigid penis somewhat uncomfortable, while others are concerned about concealment.

Inflatable penile implants are more flexible because they allow you to control the rigidity of the penis. However, they're also more expensive, more difficult to implant, and have a higher failure rate.

Luckily, recent technological and surgical improvements have reduced the incidence of mechanical failure in both types of penile implants.

It's important to remember that penile implants should be explored only when the erectile difficulties are unlikely to improve on their own, since having an implant removes the natural erection reflex. As well, penile implants won't solve sexual problems unrelated to the physical ability to have and maintain erections, such as decreased libido or psychological difficulties.

Vacuum Constriction Devices (VCD)

Note: Experts are divided about the safety and efficacy of the vacuum con-striction device. Please discuss this option with your healthcare practitioner. Vacuum constriction devices (VCD) are a non-invasive treatment option that can be used as soon as needed after surgery. Each time an erection is desired, the penis is inserted into a cylinder, and a pump is activated, either by hand or by battery. The pump causes a vacuum that draws blood into the shaft of the penis, enlarging it. Once the penis becomes erect, an elastic band or ring is placed at the base of the penis to retain the blood during intercourse. When the band is removed after intercourse, the penis returns to its previous size.

Some men and their partners enjoy building the device into the sexual experience, but others report discomfort with the disruption. Also, because of the way the erection is maintained, it isn't as sturdy as that provided by a penile implant. Again, it's up to you and your partner to decide if it works for you.

Viagra

By now, most people are away of the availability of Viagra, a relatively new drug for treating erectile dysfunction. Speak to your doctor to find out if it's an option for you. For example, Viagra may not be an option for you if you're also taking nitroglycerin. The drug's effectiveness also depends on the extent of nerve damage. For where to find more information about Viagra, see the Resources section of this book.

Injections of Vasodilatory Medication

Injections of vasodilatory medication directly into the penile shaft can stimulate or help maintain erections. The medication is called "vasodilatory" because it dilates the blood vessels in the penis, producing an erection within five to fifteen minutes. Although this may sound painful, most men report little discomfort after learning the procedure. Partners can also learn to do the injections. Erections may last up to three hours, depending on the amount of the drug injected and your response to it.

The medication most often used is prostaglandin E1 (Caverject) or a combination of papaverine and phentolamine (Regitine). Combinations of all three drugs may be the best option for long-term use and they carry a decreased risk of side effects.

While some men are quite satisfied with these drugs and experience few side effects, the long-term effects of these drugs aren't known. Many side effects have been reported, such as bruising and burning upon injection. Priapism, which is a prolonged, painful erection, has also been reported. This is a serious condition that requires immediate medical attention. Due to these concerns, some of the drugs used (such as papaverine and phentolamine) haven't been approved by the FDA for the treatment of impotence. If you're considering getting injections to treat erectile dysfunction, it's very important to speak to your doctor to determine whether it's the right option for you.

The Next Step

In general, it's best to explore the least invasive method first, and proceed from there. For example, you may wish to try medication or the vacuum device first. If these don't provide satisfactory results, you can then explore injection therapy or implants.

Remember that even if you find a treatment that works for you, your erections will probably not feel the way they did before. Aim for goals that are attainable. A realistic goal is to achieve erections that are firm enough to allow penetration.

Also, it's perfectly acceptable for you to choose no treatment to restore erections. After considering all options, you and your partner may choose not to use any of these treatment options. Although ostomy surgery may lead to erectile difficulties, it does not make orgasm impossible. In fact, some men can learn to experience orgasm without erection The added benefit of this is that it can enable you to become multi-orgasmic! Learning to experience orgasm without erection may not be an easy technique to master, and it may require that you become much more attuned to your sexual response than you were before. Nevertheless, many men find it well worth the effort. This, in combination with a little creativity and a supportive partner, can add variety to your sex life that wasn't there before. Speak to your doctor for more information, and consider requesting a referral to a sex therapist.

An expanded definition of sex helps, too. In response to cultural pressure, many men may see themselves as less masculine if they're unable to have conventional intercourse with their partners. In reality, many women enjoy manual and oral stimulation just as much as they do intercourse. Some enjoy it even more. So explore your sexuality with the help of a good sex manual, or with a sex therapist.

For gay men, the situation may be more complex. If you've had the rectum removed, the reality is that you won't be able to be the "receptive partner" during anal sex after surgery. You may benefit from exploring alternatives to anal intercourse, and you can be assured that you can still satisfy your partner. It's important, though, to never use the stoma as a receptive organ during sex – this can damage the intestine.

Body Image

Some sexual problems that appear to be physical – such as the inability to have an erection or an orgasm – may in fact be rooted in your anxiety about the changes to your body (your self-image).

The changes to your body have been considerable, and it's no wonder that you may be experiencing difficulty adjusting to them. Our social and cultural environment often downplays the importance of a man's right to experience and express emotions such as sadness, loss and grief. Men are expected to be "strong and silent," no matter how difficult the situation. But the reality is that losing bowel or urinary continence, and gaining a stoma, is not something that's easy to adjust to. Sadness, loss and grief are normal during the adjustment period, and there's nothing to be gained by ignoring their existence. One study showed that men are even more disturbed by the new self-image than are women.

It's important for you to acknowledge the changes in your body, and the emotions related to them. If you feel overwhelmed, don't hesitate to get counseling. And be assured that there's no reason for you not to have a healthy, active sex life after ostomy surgery.

Dos and Don'ts for Great Sex

And finally, here are some playful but practical "dos" and "don'ts" for great sex!

- Do enjoy baths and showers with your partner. Sex and water make for an erotic combination, and you may feel less worried about the unlikely possibility of odor or leaks if you and your partner are covered in hot, soapy water. Set the mood: candles, romantic music, and scented bath salts are all ways to increase libido. Then let your imagination run wild!

- Don't worry about the stoma getting hurt during sexplay. A small amount of bleeding is normal if the stoma gets bumped a bit. But the stoma shouldn't be used directly for sexual activity – doing this is likely to injure it, increasing the chances of prolapse and infection.
- Do dress for sex-cess in a way that makes you feel sensual and desirable. For men, this might mean a favorite pair of boxer shorts – or nothing at all. Many women enjoy donning lacy, silky lingerie. You can find lingerie that's specially designed to accommodate ostomies in publications like *The Ostomy Quarterly*. Check with your local United Ostomy Association chapter. Or you can make your own by cutting out the crotch of a silky slip, teddy or pair of underwear. Many people also buy or make attractive pouch covers, or tuck the pouch inside a belt or cummerbund.
- Do ensure that your pouch is clean, empty, and firmly adhered to your body before engaging in sex. This minimizes the chance of leaks and other intrusions on the romantic mood.
- Don't be afraid to explore alternatives to wearing a pouch during sex. Some people with sigmoid colostomies, for example, are able to wear just a colostomy plug or small pad.
- Do have a sense of humor if your ostomy should decide to participate in your lovemaking by making noises or even leaking. Passing gas – even during lovemaking – happens to almost everyone at one time or another, whether they have an ostomy or not. If it happens to you, have a chuckle about it with your partner, then get back to the business at hand.
- Do experiment with lovemaking positions. Depending on the location of the stoma, some positions may be more comfortable than others. A good sex manual helps here.
- Don't worry too much if you have occasional difficulties with sexual response, such as erections or orgasms. Women and men in relationships and individually go through periods in which sex drive may be lower than they're used to. For example, it's normal for men to experience problems achieving or maintaining an erection from time to time. If you notice a prolonged problem that's interfering with your enjoyment of sex, though, it's time to contact your doctor.
- Do include your partner in your thoughts about sexuality. Communication is important in any relationship, and even difficult situations can be opportunities to become closer to your partner. Even an ostomy leak can serve to widen the sexual horizons, if you can entice your partner into the shower or bath with you!

10
CONSIDERATIONS FOR SPECIAL GROUPS

Ostomy Care for the Elderly

If you're elderly and you have an ostomy, you probably have similar concerns about dealing with your ostomy as do people of all ages. But you may also have certain concerns about caring for your ostomy that specifically relate to the aging process.

Dealing With a New Ostomy

The prospect of undergoing surgery is an upsetting one for most people – and it can be even more so for you, if you're an older patient. In addition to all the other anxieties and fears about getting an ostomy, the difference for you might be that you see the ostomy as a threat to your independence, believing that it will keep you bedridden or overly dependent on others. Perhaps you may even consider not getting surgery at all.

The good news is that dealing with an ostomy when you're older doesn't have to be an arduous ordeal. It's just as manageable as it is for younger people, given the proper support from the healthcare professionals at your hospital. Even if you're in your eighties or nineties, it's encouraging to remember that your new ostomy can actually give you more independence than you had before.

You probably needed ostomy surgery because you were ill with cancer or other diseases of the digestive or urinary tract. Your illness itself has probably negatively affected your health and vitality. Feeling ill can be difficult emotionally as well as physically. When you're ill and feeling low, it's sometimes hard to believe that a major medical procedure like surgery can actually result in improved health.

In fact, ostomy surgery has many benefits in terms of improving health, vitality, life expectancy – and yes, even your level of independence.

If the prospect of dealing with an ostomy – changing pouches and the like – is disheartening for you, remember that most people become totally self-sufficient in terms of caring for their ostomies once the initial learning period is over. And though it may take time to learn the skills needed for ostomy care, that's what the hospital staff is there for. Before you're discharged from hospital, you can expect to have been taught basic ostomy care skills. You'll probably be scheduled for follow-up visits with your WOC nurse, as well, either at the hospital or at home, as required.

The key to eventual, successful ostomy self-care is making sure that you get the proper support. Primarily, this means getting the education you need from your WOC nurse or other hospital staff member. Here are a few tips on how to ensure that you get the support you need.

Tips for Older People with New Ostomies

1. Give yourself time to recover from surgery before you attempt to learn to care for your ostomy. If a nurse conducts an education session when you're still exhausted from surgery, you'll probably have a difficult time retaining the information. This is true for everyone, but it's especially true for you, since your body may take longer to recover from surgery than a younger person's would. If you feel that you're too exhausted to take in the information, ask the nurse if the education session can be postponed until you feel better. Many people find that sessions conducted in the morning are better than those conducted later in the day, since they feel more alert at that time.

2. Request that education sessions be conducted in an environment that's private, and that has a chair and a mirror. For example, a large bathroom with a chair and a full-length mirror may be most appropriate. The mirror is helpful because it lets you see for yourself what's happening when the nurse – and eventually you – change the appliance. If you use a wheelchair, make sure that the bathroom is large enough for you to maneuver in.

3. If you need glasses or a hearing aide, make sure that you have them and that they're in working order. Don't hesitate to request any assistance that you feel will help you learn more easily.

4. Request that the any pamphlets dealing with ostomy care be provided to you in large print format if you have trouble reading small print.

Hospitals are often able to accommodate this request for their older patients.

5. Don't hesitate to request "repeats" of an education session. It's your WOC nurse's job to make sure that you're comfortable with emptying and changing your pouch. He or she will be happy to repeat the instructions as often as needed to ensure that you're confident about managing your ostomy when you leave the hospital.

6. Once you've been discharged from the hospital, make sure that you maintain contact with your WOC nurse. This can be done via home visits if you're housebound. Use these visits to ask questions and to clear up any ostomy care issues that you're having trouble with.

7. Remember to eat well. Eating well is important for everyone, whether they are younger or older, and whether they have an ostomy or not. For many older people, though, diet is a difficult challenge. It can be hard to cook for one if you live alone, and some people find that they lose interest in food altogether. If you have an ostomy, you need to take extra care to ensure that you get adequate nutrition. Luckily, however, you don't need to worry about spending lots of money on a special diet. It's best to eat a diet high in fiber, and to drink lots of fluids. Other than that, you can just follow general dietary guidelines. If you're unsure about your diet, don't hesitate to request help. Most hospitals have a dietician on staff who can go over your diet with you and identify any areas for improvement.

8. If you feel that you won't be able to care for the ostomy at home, it may be helpful for you to bring a supportive family member – a spouse, son or daughter – with you to your education sessions, so that they can learn pouch skills as well.

If you're concerned about whether or not the pouch will show under your clothing, don't be. It's unlikely that anyone will be able to tell you have an ostomy. It's best to wait about six weeks before putting any pressure on the abdominal area, so if you prefer to wear a girdle, you should wait about this amount of time before wearing it. Keep in mind you may need to make some alterations to inner garments like girdles to accommodate the ostomy. You may also consider purchasing new undergarments specifically designed for people with ostomies. See the Resources section of this book for suggestions.

The most important thing to remember is that when you're in the learning stages, don't be afraid to ask questions about ostomy self-care.

Most people find that they often can't remember the instructions they're given the first time around because they may be too tired after surgery, or they may be emotionally distraught. Nurses are normally happy to provide instructions and information as many times as is necessary.

Handling Ostomy Care Problems

Even if you've had your ostomy for a long time and are adept at caring for it, additional health challenges related to aging can make previously easy-to-perform ostomy care tasks more challenging.

For example, many older adults who've had ostomies for many years find that they experience a fairly common problem: peristomal hernia. Peristomal hernia is an enlargement of the hole in the abdominal wall muscle that was made to bring the bowel to the skin. It happens for many reasons, the most common of which are weight gain or loss, repeated surgeries, or a less-than-ideal site for the original stoma.

The most common symptoms are the presence of a bulge around the stoma site. Most people find that, when it initially appears, the peristomal hernia is barely noticeable and doesn't cause problems with the function of the ostomy itself. If the hernia becomes enlarged (which it can due to day-to-day activities like lifting, coughing, and the like), it can make it difficult for the pouch to properly adhere to the skin.

If you're experiencing peristomal hernia, seeking medical attention for it can help reduce this type of discomfort, as well as eliminate any pouching problems it may be causing for you. Although corrective surgery is an option, in most cases the hernia is best handled by having a WOC nurse re-evaluate your pouching system to better suit your lifestyle and to eliminate any issues with incorrectly fitting appliances.

Another reason to consult your WOC nurse is if your ostomy care method is no longer working for you. For example, if you have always irrigated your colostomy, you may find that as you grow older, your manual dexterity decreases due to arthritis and other factors. This might make irrigating your colostomy difficult for you, and a simple, easy-to-use pouching system may be a better choice.

Even if you don't experience any problems with your ostomy, it's a good idea for you to consult your local WOC nurse for a re-evaluation of your ostomy care method. This is because newer products that may not have been available when you had ostomy surgery may make ostomy care much simpler for you.

Ellen, 78, who also has arthritis, has this to say about learning to manage her ostomy:

> I had been using the same appliance for years, and getting on quite well with it. But as the arthritis got worse and worse, it got harder for me to take care of the colostomy myself. It would take a long time for me to change the appliance, and it started to really bother me that I couldn't handle it as quickly as I once did. I wondered if I couldn't take care of myself, did I belong in a retirement home being taken care of? I finally talked to my doctor about it, and he put me in touch with a stoma care nurse. The nurse showed me an appliance that's much easier to deal with than the one I was using. Now that I'm able to take care of myself again without any problems, I'm only sorry that I put up with it so long before getting help.

Babies and Children with Ostomies

If you're the parent of a baby or child with an ostomy, it's likely that you were very distressed when you found out that your baby would need an ostomy. This would likely be true whether the surgery was done as an emergency or if it was elective – and possibly even more so if the ostomy was needed due to a congenital disorder. Parents may even feel guilty and fear that they have passed the disorder on to their offspring. They may also feel somewhat responsible for the "disfiguration" of their perfect baby girl or boy, and wonder what they could have done to prevent it.

But babies and children who get ostomies are likely to not only survive, but thrive. Babies as young as a few hours old undergo ostomy surgery successfully. They thrive because the ostomy allows their small bodies to absorb the nutrients they need to grow and develop – nutrients they had trouble absorbing for one reason or another before ostomy surgery. And in many cases, once the baby's body grows strong enough, surgery can be done to correct the original problem that made the ostomy necessary, and bowel continuity will be restored.

Why Do Babies and Children Get Ostomies?

Generally, babies and children who get ostomies do so because of congenital conditions, disease, or trauma.

For example, babies with Hirschprung's disease are born without certain necessary nerves (ganglia) in the descending colon, and because of this, intestinal obstruction occurs between the healthy and unhealthy parts of the colon. A typical treatment plan might be to relieve the obstruction by creating a temporary transverse colostomy, then to restore bowel continuity at a later date, once the baby's body has gained the strength necessary for corrective surgery (usually about six months to a year).

Other babies are born with defects of the spine, bowel, bladder or anus that may make either a permanent or temporary ostomy necessary.

In some cases, ostomy surgery may be elective. This is often even more difficult for the parents than emergency ostomy surgery. Because the surgery is optional, many parents are reluctant to make a decision that could "burden" their child with an ostomy temporarily or permanently.

In still other cases, the problem may not appear until the child is older. For example, for various reasons, some children experience difficulty controlling stool and urine. This can cause severe distress to the child. In most such cases, other techniques can help the child maintain continence. For example, for children with urinary incontinence, bladder massage techniques, intermittent catheterization, and medications may help. For stool incontinence, regular colonic irrigation, which is based on the same principles as colostomy irrigation, may be the answer. If all alternatives have been explored, however, elective ostomy may be the best option. In these cases, it can be very difficult for a parent to make the decision that the child needs an ostomy. It's important to keep in mind that children adjust very well to having an ostomy, and if all other options have been explored and proven fruitless, an ostomy can work perfectly well for these children.

In fact, it's often the case that children are more accepting of their ostomies than their parents are. Parents are often devastated by what they may perceive as a mutilation of their child, and fear that the child won't be able to live a normal life. These emotions can be very powerful. Luckily, support is available. Many parents find that speaking to parents who have "been there" is invaluable for providing moral support, tips on ostomy care, and sometimes just a sympathetic ear. The United Ostomy Association offers this kind of support in the form of the aptly named Parents Of Ostomy Children (POC), a group of parents with children who have undergone ostomy surgery. For information about contacting a support parent, see the Resources section of this book.

Young children, on the other hand, generally adapt quite well to their ostomies. Perhaps because they haven't yet experienced many years of life without an ostomy, they're more likely to assume that the ostomy is just part of life, something to be accepted and dealt with – and even, in some cases, shown off to friends!

Annie, now a healthy three-and-a-half-year-old, got a colostomy at four days old for Hirschsprung's Disease. One afternoon Annie was putting a makeshift pouch made from a small baggie on one of her dolls, and her best friend Jamie saw it and asked what it was. Annie showed Jamie her pouch, telling her the doctor gave it to her when she was a baby. Jamie's mother reports that her daughter came home from Annie's asking if she could "go to the doctor to get a baggie just like the one Annie has!"

Ostomy Care for Babies

Caring for an infant with an ostomy is remarkably similar to caring for an infant without one. The routines regarding diaper changing are likely to be similar to those to do with changing the ostomy pouch. There are a few things to look out for, though.

Before your baby is discharged from hospital, you should meet with your baby's hospital caregivers. Ideally, this would be a WOC nurse familiar with pediatrics or a pediatric nurse with training in ostomy care. The nurse should teach you how to care for the stoma and how to change the appliance. One-piece, extremely lightweight appliances designed especially for babies are most appropriate. A two-piece appliance is likely to be too heavy for such a small body. Don't worry about hurting your baby when you change the pouch: it's highly unlikely that changing the pouch once or twice per day will hurt your baby's skin.

It's not uncommon for an infant's stoma to change color to either a bluish or whitish shade when the baby is crying. This doesn't mean that your baby can't breathe – it happens because babies tend to pull in their knees and contract their abdominal muscles when crying, and this action temporarily traps the bowel. Once the baby stops crying, the stoma will revert to its normal red color (much like the cheek portion of the inside of your mouth).

You may want to enlist the help of a partner or other caregiver when you're changing your baby's pouch. That way, one person can entertain the baby, and hopefully prevent crying, while the other changes the pouch. It's also useful to have a simple, straightforward routine for changing the pouch. Make sure all necessary materials are assembled nearby, including a pouch with a hole cut to the correct size.

As the baby grows into a toddler, you'll need to re-fit the pouch regularly to ensure a correct fit. Eventually, a two-piece pouching system may be more appropriate, since it's easier for caregivers to manage and the baby's body is now big enough to handle it.

When your child reaches school age, be sure to discuss your child's care needs with the staff. If staff will be handling pouch changes, disposable pouches may be best. If the child prefers to change the pouch, and is old enough to handle the responsibility, a one-piece system may be easier for small hands to manage. In any case, ensure that your child has ample privacy for pouch changes, such as a private bathroom. You may also want to leave a set of "backup" appliances (pouch, adhesive, etc.) at the school, in the care of the teacher or school nurse, just in case.

It's also important that the caregiver understands that although the ostomy requires special skills to care for it, it's still perfectly manageable. Your child's ostomy should not place her or him in the position of being somehow more fragile or less capable than other children. In fact, it's often recommended that an ostomy be treated by caregivers like glasses or braces would be. Much as a child with glasses may need to remove them when playing sports, a child with an ostomy needs to consider the ostomy when taking part in different activities. What's most important is that the ostomy shouldn't prevent the child from participating in – and enjoying – the same activities as his or her classmates.

Ostomy Care for Children

For children who've had ostomies since they were babies, beginning to take care of the ostomy is a natural progression. Just as children without ostomies go through toilet training at about age two or three, children with ostomies can start taking care of their own ostomies at about that age, too. Children who don't get ostomies until toilet-training age can start to take care of the ostomy almost immediately.

To help children learn how to care for their ostomies, it's helpful to use play therapy. Play therapy lets children practice putting pouches on dolls and handling common problems. It also helps them deal with the psychological challenges of surgery. For example, ostomy supplier

Hollister distributes the Ostomy Shadow Buddy, a hospital-gowned muslin doll with wiry hair, heart-shaped eyes, and a stoma with a little ostomy pouch attached.

Children love to ask questions, and children with ostomies are no exception. They may have many questions about why they're different from other children who sit on potties rather than wear pouches. It's best to answer such questions in a simple, straightforward manner. A pamphlet available from the United Ostomy Association (UOA), called *Chris has an Ostomy*, is useful to help children learn about and deal with the ostomy. (The UOA also offers other pamphlets about children and ostomies, such as *My Child Has an Ostomy*. See the Resources section for more information

It's also useful for children to meet other children of the same age with ostomies (especially if the child was older when he or she got the ostomy). This gives both child and parents a positive role model: a child who has successfully dealt with the challenges an ostomy presents.

Even after your child has started assuming responsibility for his or her ostomy, it's still necessary for parents to keep an eye on how things are going. For example, because children grow quickly, it's necessary to check their pouches regularly and frequently for correct fit. Few things are more discouraging for a child who is learning to ostomy self-care than experiencing repeated leaks or odor despite his or her best efforts.

Children may also need to be reminded to take proper care of the stoma and the skin around it. Skin care needs for children are the same as those for any other person with an ostomy: the skin around the stoma should look just like the skin of the rest of the abdomen.

Parents can help with the learning process by making sure that a straightforward ostomy care routine is established and understood by the child, and that ostomy supplies are kept in a location that is within easy reach of the child.

It's important for children to begin taking charge of their ostomies as soon as they are able – with help from parents and other caregivers where needed, of course. Taking care an ostomy allows a child to gradually take the steps toward independence, something that's crucial for developing a healthy self-image. Ostomy self-care is really no different from any other skill a growing child learns through trial and error – whether it's tying a shoelace or learning to ride a bike without training wheels. In fact, it may be useful for parents to think of themselves as their child's "training wheels," at least as far as the ostomy is concerned. Your child definitely needs you – the training wheels – to care for the ostomy at the beginning, much as training wheels are needed when a child first climbs on a bicycle. And your help will continue to be invaluable as he or she learns ostomy self-care skills. But your child's eventual goal is to unfasten those training wheels and ride solo – and to enjoy the feeling of security and pride that comes from being self-sufficient.

Teenagers and Ostomies

If you're in your teens, you probably already have a lot on your plate. Despite the popular misconception that the teen years are footloose and fancy-free, when you're living through them, they're often anything but. There are major changes going on in your body and the intense emotions that you're experiencing can be overwhelming. Not only do you have school and sometimes work to handle, there's the upheaval of first love and the awakening of your sexuality to tackle. In short, you're trying to figure out who you are and what you want to do with your life – a tall order, at best. On top of all that, who wants to deal with an ostomy too?

Yet an ostomy is exactly what some teenagers do have to deal with. The combination of being a teenager and having an ostomy can be formidable – but then, so can being a teenager in combination with a lot of other things, too. And although it might not feel like it at the moment, overcoming this challenge and successfully learning to manage an ostomy in your teen years can build an unshakeable foundation for self-confidence and provide you with an "edge" over your peers in the topsy-turvy trip toward adulthood.

But before you can entertain such heartening thoughts for the future, you need to build a plan for successfully managing your ostomy. As a teenager with an ostomy, some of the challenges you face are similar to those of other people with ostomies, such as travel, work and diet. But you also have some unique challenges, too. Let's take a look at some practical tips that are specifically targeted to the particular challenges you face.

Talk, talk, talk – to other teens who have ostomies

Here's your chance to talk as much as you like without getting yelled at for talking in class or being on the phone all night with your friends! Unlike many older people who got their ostomies as a result of colorectal cancer, you probably had ostomy surgery due to inflammatory bowel disease: either colitis or Crohn's disease. That means you suffered – maybe for years – from all the painful and debilitating effects of IBD: diarrhea, bloating, cramps and the inability to eat normally. This may mean that you're looking forward to getting your ileostomy. You may know from talking to other teenagers that their lives improved dramatically once they were freed from IBD. In fact, it may help for you to talk to a teenager who has an ileostomy; visits can be arranged through your local chapter of the United Ostomy Association (UOA). Your visitor will probably tell you that the advantages of having an ostomy over having IBD are many: after surgery, they were able to eat what they liked, play sports and attend social activities, and travel where they wanted without worrying about the location of the nearest restroom. They'd never been able to do all these things before, and they were delighted with their newfound energy and freedom.

Visitors can also be helpful if you don't care about all these "advantages" and you're dreading ostomy surgery. It's likely that your visitor once felt the same way too, and can understand how you're feeling and sympathize with you. It's important to note, though, that after surgery is over and recovery begins, most teenagers who have ostomies are sorry only that they missed out on so much by waiting so long to get their ostomies. The UOA has an annual youth rally for 12 to 17 year-olds. If you attend, you'll find many teenagers who are only too happy to tell you about how much better their lives are now that they no longer have to contend with IBD. See the Resources section of this book for more information about the UOA's annual youth rally.

As a teenager with an ostomy, it's quite possible that you may have pelvic pouch surgery rather than conventional ileostomy surgery. Alternatives like the pelvic pouch are becoming more and more common as surgical techniques improve, and they're great because you don't have to wear an appliance. But, of course, they have their own set of problems. Bowel movements are frequent and loose, but generally settle down to become more regular and solid in the months following surgery. Pouchitis – inflammation of the lining of the pouch – can also be a very annoying problem. There are plenty of informational/support groups on the web for dealing with pelvic pouch surgery. See the Resources section of this book for more information.

Talk to your doctor or ET nurse if you have concerns about sexuality (and who doesn't?). Other sections of this book talk about how sexual function changes (or doesn't) as a result of an ostomy, but it's worth repeating that you should ask questions if you're not sure about something.

As mentioned elsewhere in this book, it's unlikely that your ostomy appliance will leak, break or smell bad. When pouches fit properly, are applied correctly and changed regularly, they rarely leak. They're unlikely to smell because most have built-in charcoal filters. But it may help for you to make a plan about what to do in case of an accidental leakage. Keep fresh pouches and an extra set of clothes, as well as some premoistened towelettes, in your locker or knapsack, and plan where you'll go to make the change (perhaps your school has a private bathroom that you can use). If you're worried about odor, include a liquid deodorizer in your "emergency kit." You can apply it to the end of your pouch to prevent odor. Some people also like to include a travel-sized can of deodorant to disperse any smell created during the emergency pouch change procedures. See the chapters on basic ostomy care and selecting an appliance for more ideas. The point is that planning how you'll handle this type of situation is useful – you won't worry about it because you'll know you can handle it.

As for gym class: if you're uncomfortable changing and showering with other students, talk to your gym teacher to find out if there are facilities that'll let you change and shower privately. You can enlist your doctor's help to do this if you're not comfortable speaking to your teacher directly.

And finally, although having an ostomy is a big adjustment, you can probably expect to start feeling more "normal" about it within a year or so. That means that although you may not like having an ostomy, you've pretty much gotten used to it, and gotten on with your life. If you're feeling like that's not true for you, then it's important to get some help. For example, if you find that you're sad or feel "flat" all the time, if you find yourself crying all the time, or if you experience continuous feelings of hopelessness, you may be depressed. Don't hesitate to talk to your parents, your doctor or a school counselor to get help.

Issues Related to Ethnicity and Culture

If you're from a minority ethnic group or culture, you may have some specific concerns related to your ostomy.

For example, if you're Muslim, you may be wondering how you can deal with the requirement to fast during Ramadan. And many cultures and religions have specific dietary requirements that need to be honored, both in the hospital and during recovery.

These concerns are all valid, and your healthcare providers need to address them. In fact, you have the right to expect your healthcare team to have awareness and understanding of the multicultural world we all live in. It's up to them to provide culturally appropriate care that respects the needs of our diverse population – no matter how unfamiliar these needs may seem to them.

That said, it's probably impossible for all healthcare providers to fully understand all the cultural and religious needs of every ethnic community. So, you may need to help educate your healthcare team about your own culture-specific needs. It's best if this education process begins right from the start, so that there's no opportunity for misunderstandings to occur.

Here's a list of information that's necessary for your healthcare team to know before beginning to treat you. Ideally, it's a good idea to communicate this information at the early stages of your treatment. For example, when you first meet with your healthcare team (doctor, WOC nurse and surgeon) you may want to bring a list of any specific needs you have. Ideally, your healthcare team will ask for this information, but it's best to have a list prepared just in case this doesn't happen. Verbally communicate the items on the list to your healthcare team or, if you prefer, provide them with a written copy.

Keep in mind that you may need to repeat this information during your hospital stay or as you're preparing to leave the hospital during your recovery period. That's another reason why it's good to keep a written list handy.

Here's a list of important information to communicate to your healthcare team:

1. Inform the healthcare team of your ethnic and religious background. For example, if your country of origin is India and your religion is Hindu, be sure to communicate this. Knowing this information helps give your healthcare providers a baseline for understanding your needs.

2. If you observe any feasts or fasts as part of your religion, explain what is required of you during these times. For example, if you observe a 12 hour fast during Ramadan, explain to your doctor or WOC nurse that you can neither eat nor drink fluids during this period. Restricting fluid intake can be difficult for your body to handle – especially if you have an ileostomy – and you need to be careful not to become dehydrated. Your doctor or WOC nurse may have some suggestions for you about dealing with fasting.

3. If you have a need to pray at specific times during the day, communicate this to your healthcare team and the hospital staff. If they understand this requirement, they can adapt hospital routine to accommodate it. For example, if your prayer involves prostration (*sujud*) you will need to make sure you wear a pouching system that is securely attached to your body.

4. If you follow the Muslim custom that the right hand is used for greeting and eating and the left for self-cleaning, then you should let your healthcare team know about this. They can provide you with a simple, one-piece appliance that is easier to manage with your left hand than a two-piece pouching system is.

5. Give your healthcare team a list of any foods that you cannot eat. For example, if you don't eat beef or if you're vegan, your hospital meals can be adapted to meet this need. You may also want to avoid gelatin, which means you won't be able to eat jelly or take any medication that has a gelatin capsule. It's particularly important that you tell your healthcare team that you can't eat gelatin, since many foods that are used to thicken output and slow bowel transit time contain it, such as marshmallows and Jell-O. Some medications in capsule form contain gelatin as well. However, if you let your healthcare team know ahead of time about your restrictions, substitutes can be provided instead.

6. If you're having trouble understanding the information being given to you due to a language barrier, request that an approved translation service be made available to you. Most hospitals keep a list of approved translation services, and it's a good idea for you to make use of one if you feel you're not understanding all the information being provided to you by your healthcare team.

7. If you have any specific needs due to your religion that affect hospital care, such as examinations and surgery, make sure you let your healthcare team know about them. For example, uncut hair is important to many Sikhs. If this is the case for you, discussing this with your doctor prior to surgery can ensure that hair removal is minimized during surgery. In addition, many Hindu, Muslim and Sikh patients prefer to be examined by members of the same sex. Let your healthcare team know if this is your preference, as well.

FINAL WORD

This book's goal was to provide you with a friendly and accessible resource on the ins and the outs of your ostomy. I've tried to cover what I believe are the most relevant topics throughout – whether what you're dealing with is a colostomy, ileostomy, urostomy or one of the continent procedures. I've also provided tips on where to go for more information so that after reading this book, you can delve further into the topics that interest you most.

I hope *Living Well with an Ostomy* has achieved this goal. Of course it's obvious that no book can tell you everything there is to know about life with an ostomy. Like most things, experience is probably the best guide of all. So I encourage you to talk to others who are experiencing the same things you are – the same challenges, and the same triumphs. No matter how alone you may feel, remember that there's someone else out there who understands. I wish you all the best that life has to offer. Cheers!

RESOURCES

The resources information is organized by topic. Each listing contains the organization's mission statement as well as its contact information. (In some cases, only the website address is provided, since some information sources are web-based only.)

Ostomy Organizations and General Information Sources

United Ostomy Association (UOA)

Mission statement
The United Ostomy Association is a volunteer-based health organization dedicated to providing education, information, support and advocacy for people who have had or will have intestinal or urinary diversions.
Contact information:
19772 MacArthur Boulevard, Suite 200
Irvine, CA 92612-2405
Tel: 1 800 826 0826
E-Mail: info@uoa.org,
Web: *www.uoa.org/*

The United Ostomy Association of Canada

Mission statement
The UOA Canada aims to inform, enlighten, connect and unite ostomates in Canada and around the world.
Contact information
United Ostomy Association of Canada Inc.

P.O. Box 825-50 Charles Street East,
Toronto, ON M4Y 2N7
Tel: 416 595 5452
Toll Free: 1 888 969 9698 - Courtesy of Hollister Limited (Canada)
Fax: 416 595 9924
E-mail:uoacan@astral.magic.ca
Web: *www.ostomycanada.ca/*

The International Ostomy Association (IOA)

Mission statement
The International Ostomy Association, an association of ostomy associations, is committed to the improvement of the quality of life of ostomates and those with related surgeries, worldwide. It provides to its member associations information and management guidelines, helps to form new ostomy associations, and advocates on all related matters and policies. The International Ostomy Association is also responsible for authoring the Charter of Ostomates' Rights.
Contact information:
Web: *www.ostomyinternational.org/*
IOA Contact Office
The British Colostomy Association has volunteered the use of its office, and members of its operational staff to the International Ostomy Association for administrative purposes. The official mailing address of IOA is:
International Ostomy Association
c/o British Colostomy Association
15 Station Road
Reading Berks RG1 1LG
England
Tel: 44 1189 391537
Fax: 44 1189 569095
Web: *www.bcass.org.uk*
E-mail: sue@bcass.org.uk

British Colostomy Association (BCA)

Mission statement
The British Colostomy Association provides support, reassurance and practical information to people with ostomies and those who

are about to have one.
Contact information
15 Station Road
Reading Berks RG1 1LG
England
Tel: 44 1189 391537
Fax: 44 1189 569095
Web: *www.bcass.org.uk*
E-mail: sue@bcass.org.uk

Wound, Ostomy and Continence Nurses Society (WOCN)

Mission statement
Founded in 1968, the Wound, Ostomy and Continence Nurses Society (WOCN) is a professional, international nursing society of more than 3,700 nurse professionals who are experts in the care of patients with wound, ostomy and continence problems.
Contact information
4700 W. Lake Ave
Glenview, IL 60025
Tel: 888 224 WOCN (toll free)
Tel: 866 615 8560
Fax: 866 615 8560
E-mail: info@wocn.org
Web: *www.wocn.org/*

OstomyWorld

Mission statement
Sponsored by ostomy supplier Hollister, this site provides information about the company's ostomy care solutions. It also provides guidelines about diet, physical activity, skin care and many other topics. You can also use the site to ask an ostomy nurse your ostomy-related questions and receive an e-mail response within 48 hours.
Contact information
Web: *www.ostomyworld.com/*

The World Ostomy Resource

Mission statement
Created "to list links to all ostomy sites in the world," this site

provides a wealth of information about all aspects of living with an ostomy.
Contact information
Web: *http://homepage.powerup.com.au/~takkenb/OstomySites.htm*

Open Directory Project – Ostomy Page

Mission statement
The Open Directory Project seeks to organize the sometimes over-whelming abundance of web-based information. This section provides a multitude of links to ostomy-related sites, including discussion groups for youth, humour pages, and inspirational stories.
Contact information
Web: *http://dmoz.org/Health/Conditions_and_Diseases/ Digestive_Disorders/Intestinal/Inflammatory_Bowel_Disease/ Ostomies/*

U.S. National Library of Medicine

Mission statement
The NLM provides access to Medline and other health information sources. It covers a wide array of topics relevant to people with ostomies, such as colorectal cancer and inflammatory bowel disease.
Contact information
Web site: *www.nlm.nih.gov/*
Colorectal cancer:
www.nlm.nih.gov/medlineplus/colorectalcancer.html
Bladder cancer:
www.nlm.nih.gov/medlineplus/bladdercancer.html
Crohn's Disease:
www.nlm.nih.gov/medlineplus/crohnsdisease.html
Ulcerative Colitis:
www.nlm.nih.gov/medlineplus/ulcerativecolitis.html
Erectile dysfunction:
www.nlm.nih.gov/medlineplus/impotence.html

The Continent Diversion Network

Mission statement
The Continent Diversion Network is a support group for people who have or plan to have an internal intestinal pouch to replace the bladder, any part of the colon, or rectum. The group publishes

a quarterly newsletter called *The Continent Connection.*
Contact information
P.O. Box 23401,
Shawnee Mission, KS 66283
Hotline: 800 456 7494
Web: *www.ostomyalternative.org/*

The J-Pouch Group

Mission statement
This site provides support and information regarding the "J-Pouch" surgical procedure, including dietary guidelines and a comprehensive Q&A.
Contact information
E-mail: webmaster@j-pouch.org
Web: *www.jpouch.org/*

Medscape

Mission statement
This website is a comprehensive resource for all medical topics, from urology to colorectal cancer. All information on the site is regularly updated, and you can register free of charge to receive a weekly newsletter telling you what's new on the site.
Contact information
WebMD Medscape Health Network
224 W. 30th Street
New York, NY 10001-5399
Tel: 212 624 3700
Web: *www.medscape.com*

Medmark (Medical Bookmarks)

Mission statement
This Web site provides links to all sorts of resources about cancer, IBD, and other health issues, including medical journals and other authoritative medical websites.
Contact information
Web: *www.medmark.org/*

Cancer

American Cancer Society

Mission statement
The American Cancer Society provides a wealth of information about all aspects of cancer, from diagnosis to treatment and rehabilitation. The website content is provided in both Spanish and English.
Contact information
Tel: 800 ACS 2345.
You can also submit an e-mail form with your question from the "Contact Us" page of the website.
Web: *www.cancer.org*

American Gastroenterological Association (AGA)

Mission statement
Billing itself as "the indispensable resource for training, education, research and patient care," the AGA is an organization of approximately 12,000 gastroenterologic physicians and scientists. The website provides links to a Public Section that contains detailed information about current research related to digestive health.
Contact information
7910 Woodmont Avenue, Suite 700
Bethesda, MD 20814
Tel: 301 654 2055
Fax: 301 654 5920
E-mail: member@gastro.org
Web: *www.gastro.org*

Bladder Cancer WebCafe

Mission statement
The Bladder Cancer WebCafe presents detailed information about current treatment options for bladder cancer, and discusses new options under investigation. It also directs users to further information on the web.
Contact information
Web: *http://blcwebcafe.org/*

CancerGuide

Mission statement
Created by cancer survivor Steve Dunn, CancerGuide's goal is to help you find answers to your questions about cancer. It's a good place to start when you're beginning your search for answers about cancer.
Contact information
Web: *http://cancerguide.org*

Cancerlinks

Mission statement
The Cancerlinks website's goal is to help you get answers to your questions about cancer by organizing the profusion of web-based information about cancer into a set of specialized topics, such as colon and bladder cancer. The site is also available in Spanish.
Contact information
Web: *www.cancerlinks.org*

Colorectal Cancer Network

Mission statement
The Colorectal Cancer Network consists of cancer survivors and their loved ones. It provides support and information to people with colorectal cancer, as well as their families and friends.
Contact information
Web: *www.colorectal-cancer.net/*

National Cancer Institute Public Inquiries Office

Mission statement
The National Cancer Institute provides explicit information about the cause, diagnosis, prevention, and treatment of cancer, as well as rehabilitation from cancer and the continuing care of cancer patients and their families. The website content is provided in both Spanish and English.
Contact information
NCI Public Inquiries Office
Suite 3036A
6116 Executive Boulevard, MSC8322
Bethesda, MD 20892-8322
Tel: To contact NCI's Cancer Information Service (CIS), in the

United States and its territories, call 800 4 CANCER (800 422 6237), Monday - Friday, 9:00 am - 4:30 pm local time. Deaf and hard of hearing callers with TTY equipment may call 800 332 8615.

Web: *www.nci.nih.gov/* or *http://cancer.gov/*

NCI also provides a live, private online assistance service Monday - Friday, 9:00 am - 7:30 pm Eastern Time. Go to *www.nci.nih.gov/contact/* and access the *LiveHelp cancer.gov* link.

New York Online Access to Health (NOAH)

Mission statement

New York Online Access to Health (NOAH) Website provides accurate, up-to-date and unbiased consumer health information in both English and Spanish.

Contact information

Cancer: *www.noah-health.org/english/illness/cancer/cancer.html*

Intestinal health and ostomy care: *www.noah-health.org/english/illness/gastro/gastro.html*

Oncolink: University of Pennsylvania Cancer Center

Mission statement

OncoLink was founded in 1994 to give cancer patients, families, healthcare professionals and the general public accurate cancer-related information at no charge. The user-friendly website is packed with information about cancer, from treatment options to coping skills. Visit their "Ask The Experts" page for specific cancer-related questions.

Contact information

OncoLink Editorial Board

University of Pennsylvania Cancer Center

3400 Spruce Street - 2 Donner

Philadelphia, PA 19104-4283

Fax: 215 349 5445

Web: *http://oncolink.upenn.edu/*

What You Need To Know About Colon Cancer

Mission statement

This site provides information about treatment options, diagnosis, support and local resources for colon cancer patients and their friends and family.

Contact information
Web: *http://cancer.about.com/cs/coloncancer/*

Crohn's Disease and Ulcerative Colitis

The Crohn's and Colitis Foundation of America Inc. (CCFA)

Mission statement
CCFA's mission is to cure and prevent Crohn's disease and ulcerative colitis through research, and to improve the quality of life of children and adults affected by these digestive diseases through education and support.

Contact information
National Headquarters - 386 Park Avenue South, 17th Floor
New York, NY 10016-8804
Tel: 212 685 3440; 800 932 2423
Fax: 212 779 4098
E-mail: info@ccfa.org
Web: *www.ccfa.org/*

Crohn's and Colitis Foundation of Canada

Mission statement
The Crohn's and Colitis Foundation of Canada (CCFC) is a national not-for-profit voluntary medical research foundation. Its mission is to find the cure for inflammatory bowel disease through research and to educate patients, their families, health professionals and the general public about IBD.

Contact information
National Office: 60 St. Clair Avenue East, Suite 600, Toronto, ON M4T 1N5
Tel: 416 920 5035; 800 387 1479,
Fax: 416 929 0364
E-mail: ccfc@ccfc.ca,
Web: *www.ccfc.ca/*

What You Need to Know About Irritable Bowel/Crohn's Disease

Mission statement
Provides ostomy-related information especially relevant for those who have ostomies as a result of IBD. Includes links to ostomy

supply companies, ostomy associations, support groups, and general information for people with ostomies. It also provides information about pelvic pouch surgery.
Contact information
Web: *http://ibscrohns.about.com/cs/ostomyinformation/*

Digestive Disease

National Institute of Diabetes and Digestive and Kidney Diseases (NIDDK)

Mission statement
Part of the National Institutes of Health, the NIDDK conducts and supports research on many of the most serious diseases affecting public health.
Contact information
General inquiries may be addressed to Office of Communications and Public Liaison, NIDDK, NIH, Building 31, Room 9A04, 31 Center Drive, MSC 2560, Bethesda, MD 20892-2560, USA.
Web: *www.niddk.nih.gov/index.htm*

Ostomy Suppliers

Coloplast North America

Mission statement
The Coloplast website offers a detailed product catalog for both conventional and continent ostomies. It contains educational resources and success stories as well as news and event updates.
Contact information
Coloplast Corporation
1955 West Oak Circle
Marietta, Georgia 30062
Tel: 800 533 0464
E-mail: gamedweb@coloplast.com
Web: *www.us.coloplast.com*

The Continent Ostomy Store

Mission statement
At the Continent Ostomy Store website, you can order supplies for your continent or conventional ostomy.
Contact information
909 Waterton Court,
Suwanee, Georgia, 30024
Tel: 866 796 0275
Fax: 770 205 5872
E-mail: ostomy@continentostomystore.com
Web: *www.continentostomystore.com/*

Convatec

Mission statement
ConvaTec is an international manufacturer of a wide variety of ostomy care and modern wound and skin care products. ConvaTec's Customer Service Department is available from 8:30 am to 5:00 pm (Eastern time) Monday to Friday.
Contact information
In the United States, ConvaTec can be contacted at the following address. See the website for international contact information.
ConvaTec
Professional Services
P.O. Box 5254
Princeton, New Jersey 08543-5254
Tel: 800 422 8811
E-mail: Professional.Services@bms.com
Web: *www.convatec.com/*
Note: Go to ConvaTec's "FAQ" page (*www.convatec.com/en_US/support/questions/index.html#request*) to learn how to order sample products and ostomy care information (such as videos and brochures).

Hollister

Mission statement
Hollister Incorporated provides ostomy care products and services in over ninety countries on six continents. In the United States, Hollister Customer Care representatives are available from 7:45 am to 4:45 pm (Central time) Monday through Friday.

Contact information
Hollister Inc.
Customer Care Department
2000 Hollister Drive
Libertyville, Illinois 60048
Tel: 800 323 4060
Web: *www.hollister.com/*

Nu-Hope Laboratories

Mission statement
A long-time designer and manufacturer of ostomy equipment and supplies, Nu-Hope Laboratories develops specialty and custom ostomy products as well as pouches and support belts. The website includes a product catalog and a "Workshops" page that contains how-to information about using ostomy supplies.
Contact information
Nu-Hope Laboratories, Inc.
P.O Box 331150
Pacoima, California 91333-1150
Tel: 800 899 5017
Fax: 818 899 2079 or alternately 818 899 7711
E-mail: Info@Nu-Hope.com
Web: *www.nu-hope.com/*

Medical Care Products Inc.

Mission statement
An active UOA chapter member in Jacksonville, Florida, Medical Care Products, Inc. carries a complete line of ostomy supplies. A registered nurse is part of the staff and is available to answer your questions.
Contact information
Medical Care Products Inc.
P.O. Box 10239
Jacksonville, FL
32247-0239
Tel: 904 396 7827 (local); 800 741 0110 (toll free)
Fax: 904 396 7829
Web: *www.ostomymcp.com*

Turnstone Products Inc.

Mission statement
Creators of OSTI-WEAR undergarments, Turnstone Products' website showcases the different styles of undergarments – from panties to boxers – that are made especially for men and women with ostomies.
Contact information
Turnstone Products, Inc.
545 Mingarry Drive, Richmond Hill,
GA 31324
Tel: 912 727 4822
Web: *www.ostiwear.com/*

Ostomies and Children

Parents of Ostomy Children (POC)

Mission statement
POC welcomes and supports children and families. POC continues to develop a support network of trained visitors across the country, updates its resource list, and provides educational and social opportunities at the UOA Annual Conference.
Contact information
See the UOA contact information.
Web: *www.uoa.org/poc.html*

Shadow Buddies and the Shadow Buddies Foundation

Mission statement
Created by the mother of a child with an ostomy, Shadow Buddies help children and their families cope with their illness or disease by letting them know that it's okay to be a little different. Each doll is customized to have the same illness as that of the child who receives it. The dolls are inexpensive and can be ordered through the website or by calling the toll-free number below.
Contact information
Shadow Buddies and the Shadow Buddies Foundation
10680 Barkley,
Suite 210

Overland Park, Kansas 66212
Tel: 913 642 4646; 888 BUDDIES (toll-free)
Fax (913) 642-4233
Web: *www.shadowbuddies.com/buddybook/*

Ostomies and Sexuality

The Cancer Supportive Care Web Site

Mission statement
Created by medical professionals, the Cancer Supportive Care Web Site provides information about sexuality and intimacy as they relate to cancer diagnoses. Links to other sources of information and a suggested reading list are provided.
Contact information
Cancer Supportive Care Web Site
1708 B MLK, Jr Way
Berkeley, CA
94709
E-mail: support@cancersupportivecare.com
Tel: 510 649 8177
Fax: 510 649 8276
Web: *www.cancersupportivecare.com/sexuality.html*

Information About Viagra

Contact information
VIAGRA Consumer Automated Helpline: 888 4VIAGRA
VIAGRA Consumer Information: 888 733 2009
Web: *www.viagra.com/*

Information About Erectile Dysfunction

Mission statement
Discusses many different treatments for erectile dysfunction, including Viagra.
Contact information
Web: *www.seekwellness.com/impotence/index.htm*

Bladder Cancer WebCafe – Impotence Guide

Mission statement

The Bladder Cancer WebCafe presents detailed information about current treatment options for bladder cancer, and discusses new options under investigation. It also directs users to further information on the web.

Contact information

Web: *http://blcwebcafe.org/impotenceguide.asp*

GLOSSARY

Note: This list is not exhaustive. These are not literal dictionary definitions, but rather definitions created solely for the context of this book.

Acidophilus: Acidophilus supplements are often used to prevent or treat uncomplicated diarrhea caused by disruptions in the normal balance of intestinal flora. They can be purchased at most health food stores.

Appliance accessories are products that may be used to enhance the performance of your pouching system. Examples are belts, pouch covers, skin wipes, cleansers and skin barriers.

Aromatherapy: Aromatherapy is a healing therapy that asserts that essential oils (the pure, distilled aromatic oils of specific plants) can help promote the health of both body and mind.

Barrier openings are defined by the pre-cut hole in the skin barrier. It's usually the same size as the stoma, but should not be smaller than the diameter of the stoma.

Bedside or night drainage collection systems are large collection bags for urine. A person with a urostomy connects the appliance to a bedside drainage collection system at night. Also known as a bedside drainage systems.

Blockage: Blockage results when an incompletely digested piece of food fails to exit the body properly through the stoma, or when scar tissues from previous surgery constrict the bowel. Blockages can occur anywhere in the intestinal tract. They're sometimes treatable at home, though some of the more severe cases may mean a trip to the hospital. Also called intestinal obstruction.

Brooke ileostomy: The standard, conventional type of ileostomy surgery. The ileum is brought to the surface of the abdomen and a stoma is created. Also called a conventional ileostomy.

Chlorophyll: Chlorophyll is the green pigment that plants use to convert solar energy for photosynthesis. Chlorophyll is used to reduce the odor of bad breath, urine and feces. Dietary sources of chlorophyll include algae, barley grass, chlorella, spirulina, wheat grass and dark green leafy vegetables. It's available in powder form from many health food stores.

Closed-end appliances are appliances that are not drainable from the bottom. When this type of appliance needs to be emptied, it's removed and thrown away. Typically, people with colostomies use closed-end appliances.

Colon: Another term for the large intestine or last portion of the gastrointestinal tract.

Colonic conduits, like ileal conduits, are a type of urostomy or urinary diversion. A portion of the colon is used as a passageway (conduit) to allow urine to exit the body. The urine flows from the kidneys, down the ureters, through the conduit and out the stoma.

Colorectal cancer: Cancer that occurs in the colon and rectum. Colon and rectal cancers often begin as polyps (small clumps of cells). Over time some of these polyps become cancerous, leading to colorectal cancer.

Colostomy irrigation: Colostomy irrigation involves the use of special colostomy irrigation equipment to evacuate stool into the toilet. It's similar to a self-conducted enema that keeps the bowel stool-free for up to 72 hours (although most people find that 24 to 48 hours is the norm).

Colostomy reversal: Temporary colostomies are created to remove/bypass diseased portions of the colon and give the healthy portions time to heal from surgery. The operation that takes place to reconnect the healthy portions of the colon is called a colostomy reversal. Also known as a colostomy closure.

Colostomy: A surgically created opening in the abdominal wall into the large intestine or colon. A colostomy can occur at any point along the length of the colon. Where the ostomy is located – and what it's called – depends on what part of the colon is affected. The most common type of colostomy is the sigmoid colostomy; other types include ascending, transverse, and loop colostomies. Colostomies may be temporary or permanent. Temporary colostomies may be required after bowel surgery, to give a portion of the bowel a chance to rest and heal. Once healing is complete, the colostomy can be reversed or closed, and normal bowel function restored. Permanent colostomies are necessary when disease affects the end part of the colon.

Congenital abnormality: A health abnormality that is present at birth or genetically inherited. Familial Polyposis (FAP) is an example of a congenital abnormality. Also known as a birth defect.

Continent intestinal reservoir: This type of ileostomy consists of a reservoir inside the abdomen. The stoma is small and flush with the skin, and the reservoir stores waste until it's emptied using a catheter two to four times per day. Also called the Koch pouch after the surgeon who introduced it.

Convexity in an appliance is the outward (convex) curving of the portion of the appliance that has contact with the skin, usually the skin barrier. Convex appliances can be useful if the skin around the stoma is irritated because the stoma is short, flush with the skin, or retracted. The convex shape provides form to the skin barrier and support to the peristomal skin.

Crohn's disease: An inflammatory bowel disease, Crohn's disease is characterized by chronic ulceration of any part of the gastrointestinal tract, from the mouth to the anus. Medication and surgery cannot cure Crohn's disease, though they may help relieve symptoms.

Cut-to-fit barriers are barriers that need to be cut before they're applied to the body. A cut-to-fit barrier is suitable directly after surgery, when the stoma is still changing sizes, or if the shape of the stoma is not round.

Dermatitis: Dermatitis is an inflammation of the skin that produces itching, flaking, scaling and sometimes color changes. In many cases, dermatitis is the result of allergies to substances like creams, ointments, rubber or latex.

Distal stoma: On a double barrel colostomy, the distal stoma is the stoma that's closest to the end of the gastrointestinal tract. Since it's no longer connected to the digestive system, it does not produce stool, though it can produce mucous. Also known as a mucous fistula, it can be formed at a site separate from the proximal colostomy.

Diverticulitis: Diverticulitis is characterized by the inflammation of the mucous membranes of the colon. This inflammation occurs in small, pouch-like areas called diverticula in the colon. Once formed, these diverticula don't go away. Diverticula can become inflamed if waste matter becomes trapped in them, leading to symptoms such as fever, chills and pain. Colostomy surgery may be performed if these symptoms are severe and long-lasting.

Drainable appliances are appliances that open from the bottom to empty the contents. A drainable appliance requires some type of clamp on the bottom to keep it closed. Typically, people with colostomies or ileostomies use drainable appliances.

Familial Adenomatous Polyposis (FAP) is a hereditary disease, the symptoms of which are polyps (abnormal lumps of cells). If one parent has the gene for FAP, each child has a 50 percent chance of inheriting it. All children who inherit the gene will develop colorectal cancer in adulthood, if FAP is left untreated. However, overall, FAP is responsible for only one percent of colorectal cancer.

Filters are charcoal vents in an ostomy appliance that allow gas to escape and be deodorized. Filters can be constructed as part of the appliance's film, as in a closed appliance, or they may be replaceable, as in a drainable appliance.

Flanges are the plastic rings on a two-piece pouching system. The flange on the pouch and the flange on the skin barrier must match to create a well-fitted pouching system.

Gastroenterologist: A gastroenterologist is a medical doctor who specializes in treating diseases of the gastrointestinal (digestive) tract.

Hirschsprung's disease is a congenital (present at birth) abnormality characterized by obstruction of the colon. Inadequate muscular movement of the bowel due to missing nerves (ganglia) causes this obstruction, and stool cannot exit the body. Corrective ostomy surgery provides a way for stool to exit the body.

Homeopathy: Based on the premise that like cures like, homeopathic medicines use minute doses of substances that cause specific symptoms in a healthy person to alleviate those same symptoms in a person who is ill. Healthcare practitioners such as naturopaths and some medical doctors incorporate homeopathy into their medical treatment plans.

Ileal conduit is the most common type of urostomy. Also called the ileal loop or Bricker's loop after the surgeon who developed the procedure, it involves using a segment of ileum (small intestine) to create a passageway to divert urine. The urine flows from the kidneys, down the ureters, through the conduit and out the stoma.

Ileoanal reservoir (or ileoanal pouch anastomosis): An internal pouch formed from small intestine. The pouch provides a storage space for stool. The pouch is often "J" shaped, but it can be "W" or "S" shaped as well. For this surgery to be possible, the anal sphincter muscles must still be intact. Stool is passed through the anus. This provides lifestyle benefits over ileostomies, though stool is often loose and frequent (four to six times per day and one or two times per night). Also known as a pelvic pouch. Only possible in patients with ulcerative colitis or FAP.

Ileostomy: A surgically created opening in the abdominal wall into the small intestine. The end of the ileum (the lowest part of the small intestine) is brought through the abdominal wall to form a stoma. An ileostomy may be performed when a diseased or injured colon cannot be treated successfully with medication. The conventional Brooke ileostomy is still the standard and the most common type of ileostomy.

Ileorectal anastomosis: Ileorectal anastomosis is a type of surgery that joins the ileum with the rectum. Surgery involves the removal of the entire colon. The rectum is left in place, and the small bowel is attached to it. This type of surgery is possible in patients with ulcerative colitis, Crohn's disease and cancer.

Ileum: The last section of the small intestine before it connects to the colon.

Imperforate anus: A relatively common congenital abnormality that occurs in about 1 out of 5,000 infants, imperforate anus is characterized by the absence or obstruction of the anal opening. The rectum or the colon may be connected to the vagina in girls or to the urethra, bladder, base of the penis or scrotum in boys. Normal elimination can become possible with surgery, including ostomy surgery.

Inflammatory bowel disease (IBD) is a term used to describe two chronic intestinal disorders: Crohn's disease and ulcerative colitis. Both Crohn's disease and ulcerative colitis cause abdominal pain, cramping, fatigue and diarrhea.

Internal continent reservoir: Internal continent reservoirs are alternatives to traditional urostomies. They involve the creation of pouches and outlets from parts of gastrointestinal organs, usually portions of small intestine or the colon. A catheter is used to drain urine from the pouch through an abdominal stoma. Examples of internal continent reservoirs are the Koch, Indiana, Mainz, Miami, Studer, and Mitrofanoff pouches.

Intravenous (IV) tube: During surgery, an intravenous tube is attached to a vein in your hand or arm. The IV provides you with fluid and medications during the operation and directly afterward, until your digestive system starts working again.

Leg bag: A collection bag for urine that is larger than a regular urostomy pouch. It may be useful while traveling, when rest stops are infrequent.

Mucous fistula: On a double barrel colostomy, the mucous fistula is the stoma that's closest to the end of the gastrointestinal tract. Since it's no longer connected to the digestive system it produces mucous rather than stool. Also known as a distal stoma.

One-piece appliances are composed of a skin barrier and pouch that are already attached to one another. They're applied in a one-step application to the skin. Most one-piece appliances don't include a plastic ring or flange.

Opaque appliances are colored as opposed to transparent, so that the contents of the appliance aren't visible.

Ostomy: An ostomy (or stoma) is an artificial opening between a cavity and the surface of the body.

Parastomal hernias are hernias near the stoma. A fairly common problem, they occur when a bulge or tear in the abdominal muscle allows an organ or tissue to squeeze through. They may occur if the abdominal wall opening becomes larger than the stoma, allowing another loop of bowel to slip through and causing a bulge around the stoma. Parastomal hernias usually aren't serious, but it's worth consulting your WOC nurse for evaluation – especially if you're having trouble with your appliance as a result of the hernia (your WOC nurse can work with you to select a more appropriate appliance).

Peristomal skin is the skin directly surrounding the stoma.

Polyps: Polyps are abnormal clumps of cells that form in the colon or rectum, or both. These clumps are mushroom-shaped and grow on the inside lining of the colon. Polyps are common in individuals with Familial Polyposis, though they are also quite common in people over 50 years old. Most polyps are small (measuring less than one centimeter), but some measure three centimeters or more.

Pouches are bags that collect the discharge from the ostomy. Also known as appliances or pouching systems.

Pouchitis: Pouchitis is a condition in which the mucosa, or lining, of an internal pouch becomes inflamed. It can be a long-term problem for some, but most cases can be cleared up with antibiotics. Symptoms include a steadily increasing stool frequency (up to eight or more per day), bleeding, abdominal cramping, fever, and an urgent need to defecate.

Prolapse, or "falling out," occurs when the stoma becomes longer. This may happen during pregnancy, or weak abdominal muscles may cause it.

Proximal stoma: On a double barrel colostomy, the proximal stoma is the stoma that's nearest to the upper gastrointestinal tract. It provides a way for stool to exit the body.

Retraction occurs when scar tissue pulls the stoma inward toward the body. Retraction may make getting a good seal for your appliance difficult, because the stool may slip under the wafer. Sometimes a convex insert or appliance alleviates this problem.

Sitz bath: Sitz baths can help reduce inflammation and pain (such as that caused by surgical incision in the perineal region) by increasing the blood flow to the pelvic and abdominal areas. To prepare a sitz bath, fill a tub or basin so that the water covers the hips and reaches the middle of the abdomen. Sitz baths can use hot or cold water only, or they can alternate between the two, depending on their purpose. Consult your doctor or WOC nurse for more information.

Skin barriers are products placed on the body for the purpose of protecting the skin. Skin barriers are adhesive, but have different properties based upon formulation.

Spina bifida: Spina bifida is a congenital disorder characterized by incomplete development of the brain, spinal cord, or their protective coverings. Infants born with spina bifida may also have bowel and bladder complications that require corrective ostomy surgery.

Stoma: During surgery, an opening is created in the abdomen and a portion of the small or large intestine is brought through the abdominal wall. This is called the stoma. The stoma allows the release of waste from the body. Most people wear appliances over the stoma to collect the waste, although some choose other methods of stoma management, such as irrigation.

Stool: The term used to describe waste material released from the bowel.

Total parenteral nutrition (TPN): A complete form of nutrition that's administered via an intravenous infusion.

Transparent appliance: The film on this type of appliance is designed to allow you to see the contents. Transparent appliances are useful in some circumstances, such as directly after surgery when nurses need to ensure that your ostomy is working well.

Two-piece appliances include a skin barrier with flange and a pouch with flange. The two flanges lock together to create the pouching system.

Ulcerative colitis: An inflammatory bowel disease, ulcerative colitis is a chronic condition in which the mucous membrane of the colon becomes inflamed and develops ulcers, causing gas, bloating, pain, and bloody diarrhea. Ulcerative colitis can range from mild to severe. The disease can be completely eliminated by surgically removing the colon.

Urinalysis: A urinalysis is a chemical examination of the urine with the goal of detecting abnormalities such as urinary tract infections, renal disease, and diseases of other organs that result in abnormal metabolites (break-down products) appearing in the urine.

Urinary tract infection (UTI): An infection that typically involves the kidneys or bladder. Some warning signs of a urinary tract infection include dark cloudy urine, strong smelling urine, back pain, fever, loss of appetite, nausea and vomiting.

Urologist: A medical doctor who specializes in treating diseases of the urinary tract.

Urostomy appliance: This type of appliance has a drain valve or spout at the end since it's designed to drain liquid contents (usually urine). A person with a urostomy or urinary diversion would use this type of appliance.

Urostomy: A urostomy, or urinary diversion, is a surgically created opening that allows urine to flow out of the body. Typically, a urostomy is created when the bladder is either not functioning or has to be removed. There are several different types of surgeries, but the most common are ileal conduit and colonic conduit.

Wound ostomy continence (WOC) nurses specialize in the care of people who have wound, ostomy or continence concerns. Also known as an enterostomal therapy (ET) nurse.

BIBLIOGRAPHY

About.com. "Inflammatory Bowel Disease 101." <*ibscrohns.about.com/library/weekly/aa050600a.htm*>

About.com. "Ten tips for recovering from abdominal surgery." <*ibscrohns.about.com/library/weekly/aa030101a.htm*>

American Gastroenterological Association. "Colorectal Cancer Detection and Prevention." <www.gastro.org/public/crc.html>

American Gastroenterological Association. "What is a gastroenterologist?"<*www.gastro.org/public/definition.html*>

American Gastroenterological Association. "Inflammatory bowel disease." <*www.gastro.org/public/ibd.html*>

Balch, James F. and Phyllis A. Balch. *Prescription for Nutritional Healing*, Second Edition. (Garden City Park, New York: Avery Publishing Group, 1997.)

Ball, Edna M., RN, MEd. "A Teaching Guide for Continent Ileostomy." (Ostomy Guide, Part Two). *RN* (Volume 63 December, 2000. 35-36, 38, 40, 42).

Bekkers, M.J.T., A.M. Dulmen, W. Van Den Borne and G.P. Van Berge Henegouwen. "Survival and Psyhosocial Adjustment to Stoma Surgery and NonStoma Bowel Resection: A 4-year Followup". *Journal of Psychosomatic Research* (Volume 42, Ni. 3, pp. 235-244, 1997).

Black, Patricia K. 2000. *Holistic Stoma Care*. (London: Harcourt Publishers Limited, 2000.)

Black, Patricia. "Practical Stoma Care". *Nurs Stand* (Volume 14[41] June 28, 2000.47-55).

Bladder Cancer Café. "Internal Pouches - Continent Reservoirs." *<blcwe-bcafe.org/internalpouches.asp>*

Cancerfacts.com. "About Colostomy Surgery." *<www.cancerfacts.com>*

Colorectal Cancer Network. "What is colorectal cancer?" *<www.colorectal-cancer.net/questions.htm>*

Convatec Connection. "Continent Ileostomy - Surgical Alternative." *<www.convatec.com/en_GB/education/what_is/whatIsRepository/ileostomystudy.html>*

Convatec Connection. "Colostomy." *<www.convatec.com/en_US/education/what_is/whatIsRepository/colostomystudy.html>*

Convatec Connection. "Ileostomy." *<www.convatec.com/en_GB/education/what_is/whatIsRepository/ileostomystudy.html>*

Crohn's and Colitis Association of America. "Standard Ileostomy." *<www.ccfa.org/medcentral/library/surgery/ileostom.htm>*

Crohn's and Colitis Foundation of America. "Alternatives To The Standard Ileostomy." *<www.ccfa.org/medcentral/library/ surgery/altileo.htm>*

Crohn's and Colitis Foundation of America. "Before & After Surgery." *<www.ccfa.org/medcentral/library/surgery/surg2a.htm>*

Crohn's and Colitis Foundation of America. "Pouchitis." *<www.ccfa.org/medcentral/library/surgery/pouch2a.htm>*

Crohn's and Colitis Foundation of Canada. "Sexuality, Fertility, Pregnancy and Inflammatory Bowel Disease."*<www.ccfc.ca/en/info/brochures/sexuality.html>*

Dorr Mullen, Barbara. *The Ostomy Book.* (Palo Alto, California: Bull Publishing Co., 1992.)

Fetrow, C.W., PharmD and Juan R Avila. PharmD. *Professional's Handbook of Complementary and Alternative Medicines*, Second Edition. (Springhouse, Pennsylvania: Springhouse, 2001.)

Flagg, Marianne. "Ileoanal or ileorectal anastomosis." WebMD. Last updated: August 31, 2001.

Garbee, Deborah Delaney. RN, MN, CNOR and Judith A Gentry, APRN, MSN, OCN. "Coping with the Stress of Surgery." *AORN J* (Volume 73(5) May 2001.946, 949-951).

Hale, Barbara and Vicki Fong. "Vitamin D Deficiency and Bowel Diseases Connected." April 18, 2000. Pennsylvania State University. <*www.psu.edu/ur/2000/vitamind.html*>

Hobbs, Christopher. *Herbal Remedies for Dummies.* (Foster City, California: IDG Books Worldwide, 1998.)

Hull, Tracy L. MD. "Surgical Management Of Crohn's Disease." The Cleveland Clinic Foundation, Department of Colorectal Surgery. Cleveland, Ohio. <*www.fascrs.org/coresubjects/1999/crohns/crohns.html*>

Hurd, Linda B. RN, MSN. "An Overview of Ileoanal Reservoir (Pouch) Surgery." The J-Pouch Group, 1997-2002. <*www.j-pouch.org/Whatis.html*>

IOA Coordination Committee. "The Ostomates' Bill of Rights." International Ostomy Association. Created June 1993, revised June 1997. <*www.ostomyinternational.org/aboutus.htm#rights*>

Jeter, Katherine F. *These Special Children.* (Palo Alto, California: Bull Publishing Company, 1982.)

Joachim, Gloria RN, MSN and Sonia Acorn, RN, Ph.D. "Stigma of visible and invisible chronic conditions." *J Adv Nursing.* (Volume 32 [1] July, 2000.243-248.)

Katz, Joshua, MD. "Stoma Surgery: Trying To Get It Right." The Cleveland Clinic Florida, Department of Colorectal Surgery. Weston, Florida. <*www.geocities.com/broward_ostomy/Article_5.html*>

Keville, Kathi. *Aromatherapy for Dummies.* (Foster City, California: IDG Books Worldwide, 1999.)

Lacroix, A. "Patient's Experiences with their disease: learning from the difference and sharing common problems." *Patient Education and Counseling.* (Volume 26 1995.301-312.)

Matthews, Shirley D. MSN, RN, CWOCN; Courts, Nancy Fleming Ph.D., RN. "Orthotopic Neobladder Surgery: Nursing care promotes independence in patients with bladder cancer." *American Journal of Nursing.* (Volume 101 [7] July 2001 pp 24AA-24GG.)

Mayo Foundation for Medical Education and Research *Polyps of the Colon and Rectum.*(Mayo Clinic Rochestor. 1996-2002.)

Medbroadcast.com. "What is inflammatory bowel disease?"*<www.med-broadcast.com/health_topics/health_conditions/inflammatory_bowel/index.s html?gas_i_whatis.html>*

Mount Sinai Hospital. "A Guide for Families with Familial Adenomatous Polyposis." *<www.mtsinai.on.ca/familialgican/FAPEnglish/fap.html>*

National Cancer Institute. "Colon and Rectal Cancer Home Page." <http://www.nci.nih.gov/cancer_information/cancer_type/colon_and_rectal/>

National Library of Medicine. *Medline Medical Encyclopedia.* *<www.nlm.nih.gov/medlineplus/encyclopedia.html>*

Northwestern Memorial Hospital – Nutrition Services. *Ostomy Diet Guidelines.* (Northwestern Memorial Hospital: May, 2001.)

Northwestern Memorial Hospital – Nutritional Support Department of Pharmacy. *Total Parenteral Nutrition: Discharge Instructions.* (Northwestern Memorial Hospital: October, 1999.)

Northwestern Memorial Hospital – Surgical Nursing with the Ambulatory Surgery Unit. *A Patient Guide To Surgery.* (Northwestern Memorial Hospital: January, 2001.)

Northwestern Memorial Hospital – Wound, Ostomy and Continence Nurses. *A Patient Guide to Colostomy Care.* (Northwestern Memorial Hospital: June, 2001.)

Northwestern Memorial Hospital – Wound, Ostomy and Continence Nurses. *A Patient Guide to Ileostomy Care.* (Northwestern Memorial Hospital: June, 2001.)

Northwestern Memorial Hospital –Wound, Ostomy and Continence Nurses. *A Patient Guide to Urinary Diversions.* (Northwestern Memorial Hospital: June, 2001.)

O'Brien, Bridget K. BSN, RN, CWOCN. *Coming of Age with an Ostomy.* (Lippincott Williams & Wilkins, Inc. Volume 99 [8] August 1999. 71-74, 76.)

Phillips, Robert H., Ph.D. *Coping with an Ostomy.* (Wayne, New Jersey: Avery Publishing Group Inc., 1986.)

Rosenthal, Sara. *The Gastrointestinal Sourcebook.* (Lincolnwood, Illinois: Lowell House Publishing Group, 1998.)

Schover, Leslie, Ph.D. *Sexuality and Fertility After Cancer.* (New York: John Wiley & Sons, 1997.)

Shelton, Brenda K. MS, RN, CCRN, AOCN. "Intestinal Obstruction." *AACN Clinical Issues: Advanced Practice in Acute & Critical Care* (Volume 10 [4)] November 1999.478-491.)

Silberman, Sara M. *Coping With Your Fear of Surgery.* Crohn's and Colitis Foundation of Canada. <*http://www.ccfa.org/news/previous/surgfeat.htm*>

Spencer, Michael P, MD, FACS, FASCRS. "Ostomies and Stomal Therapy." American Society of Colon and Rectal Surgeons. Department of Surgery, University of Minnesota, Minnesota, Minneapolis. <*www.fascrs.org/coresubjects/ostomies_stomal_therapy.html*>

SpringNet for Nurses. "Troubleshooting skin complications." <*www.springnet.com/ce/p105bs03.htm*>

Texas Pediatric Surgical Associates. "Hirschsprung's Disease (Aganglionic Megacolon)." <*www.pedisurg.com/PtEduc/Hirschprung's_Disease.htm*>

Texas Pediatric Surgical Associates. "Imperforate Anus." <*www.pedisurg.com/PtEduc/Hirschprung's_Disease.htm*>

The Canadian Association for Enterostomal Therapy (CAET). *A Guide to Living with a Colostomy.* (Ottawa, Ontario: 1996.)

The Canadian Association of Enterostomal Therapy (CAET). *A Guide to Living with an Ileostomy.* (Ottawa, Ontario: 1998.)

The Canadian Association of Enterostomal Therapy (CAET). *A Guide to Living with an Urostomy.* (Ottawa, Ontario: 1998.)

The Canadian Association of Enterostomal Therapy (CAET). *A Guide to Living with a Colostomy.* (Ottawa, Ontario: 1998.)

The StayWell Company. "Living with your urostomy: A Guide to Self-Care." The StayWell Company, 1999.

The United Ostomy Association of Canada. *Young Person's Guide To Living with an Ostomy.* (July, 2001.)

Thompson, Julia, RN, BSN, CETN. "Part One: A Practical Ostomy Guide." *RN* (Volume 63 [11] November 2000.61-64, 66, 68.)

Ullman, Dana, M.PH. *The Consumer's Guide to Homeopathy*. (New York: The Putnam Berkley Group, 1995.)

UMHS. "Department Of Surgery Clinical Programs: Continent Ileostomy." <www.med.umich.edu/surg/gen/Ileostomy.htm>

United Ostomy Association of Canada. *Ostomy: A Reference Guide*. (The United Ostomy Association of Canada, 1998.)

United Ostomy Association of Canada. *Travel Tips for Ostomates*. (Ostomy Resource Center, Mount Sinai Hospital, Toronto, ON Canada.)

United Ostomy Association, Inc. "Colostomy Fact Sheet." Irvine, CA. <*www.uoa.org*>

United Ostomy Association, Inc. "Ileostomy Fact Sheet." Irvine, CA. <*www.uoa.org*>

United Ostomy Association, Inc. "Urostomy Fact Sheet." Irvine, CA. <*www.uoa.org*>

University of Wisconsin Department of Surgery. "Ileal Pouch Reconstruction." University of Wisconsin, 2000. <*http://www.surgery.wisc.edu/*>

UPMC Health System. *Care of Stoma*. (UPMC Health System, Pittsburgh, PA: 2000.)

UPMC Health System. *Ostomy Nutrition Guide: Information for Patients*. (UPMC Health System, Pittsburgh, PA. 2000.)

Vaccari, Joy, RN, BSN, CETN. "Certain Drugs May Not Work In Ileostomy Patients." *RN*. (Volume 62 [2] February 1999.69.)

Weekakoon, Patricia. "Sexuality and the patient with a stoma." *Sexuality and disability*. (Volume 19, Number2, Summer 2001.)

White, Craig, BSc. ClinPsyD, PGCCT, CPsychol. "Psychological Management of Stoma-related Concerns." *Nurs Stand*. (Volume 12 [36]. May 27-June3, 1998.35-38.)

World Ostomy Resource. <*http://homepage.powerup.com.au/~takkenb/OstomySites.htm*>

Wright, Kathleen Dredge. "Colostomy." *Gale Encyclopedia of Medicine*. (Gale Research, 1999.)

INDEX

A

Activities, see Lifestyle
Anus, 30
   see also Colostomy, about
Appliances (pouching systems), 71-72
   accessories, 73
   Brooke ileostomies and, 69
   closed-ended, 71-72
   drainable, 72
   emptying and changing, 74-76
   J-pouch, 32
   ostomy suppliers, 150-153
   other how-to's, 76-77
   types of ostomies and, 69-70
   WOC nurse as resource, 71
Aromatherapy, pre-surgery, 50
   post-surgery, 58-59
   see also Homeopathy
Associations, 141-155
   United Ostomy Association, 141
   The United Ostomy Association of
      Canada, 141
   The International Ostomy
      Association, 142

B

Babies, see Children and Babies
Bladder, bladder cancer website, 155
   cancer of, 37
   infections, 59-60
   substitute, 39
   see also Urostomies
Bleeding, IBD and, 23
   medications and, 77
   stoma and, 77

Blockage (intestinal obstruction), 83
   prevention of, 83-84
Body image, 105
   adjusting to new, 105-106, 122
   emotional recovery and, 113-114
   men and, 117, 122
   women and, 113-114
Bowels, 67-68
   see also Blockage
Brooke ileostomy,
   see Appliances and Ileostomy,
      types of

C

Caffeine, 33,81
Cancer, resources and information,
     146-149
   see also Colorectal cancer
Care of ostomy, 63-64
Charter of Rights, see Ostomate's rights
Children and babies, 129-131
   ostomy care for babies, 131-132
   ostomy care for children, 132-134
   support groups and associations, 153
   see also Teenagers
Colitis, See Ulcerative colitis and
      Inflammatory bowel disease
Colonic conduit, see Conduit
Colorectal cancer, risk factors for, 19
   symptoms of, 19
   treatment of, 19-20
   see also Familial adenomatous
      polyposis
Colostomy, 25-26
   basic care and management of,
      65-68

irrigation, 66-67
permanent, 29
stoma plug, 68
surgical reversal, 30
temporary, 30
types of, 27-29
Conduits, 39, 46
see also Urostomies
Congenital conditions, 18, 129-131
Constipation, 88
pain medication as cause of, 96
stool softeners, 96
laxatives, 96
Continent ileostomy, 32-37
continent intestinal reservoir (Koch
pouch), 34-35
Crohn's disease, 21
resources and information, 149-150
see also Inflammatory bowel disease
Cultural and ethnicity issues, 136-138

D

Dehydration, ileostomies and, 31
treatment of, 89-91
Deodorants, see Odor
Descending colostomy, 29
Diarrhea, acidophilus as treatment for,
89
causes of, 88-89
foods to avoid during, 89
Gatorade-like drink recipe, 90
Diet and nutrition, 80
bowels and, 67-68
caffeine, 33, 81
diabetes and, 80
foods, potentially problematic,
84-85, 87, 89
guidelines for, 80-82
inflammatory bowel disease and, 22
ileostomy and, 90-91
minimizing odor and gas with,
84-88
potassium and sodium, sources of,
91
see also Blockage

Digestive system, diagram, 26
digestive disease information, 150
see also Bowels and Diet and nutrition
Diverticulitis, 26

E

Elderly and ostomies, 125-129
Emotions, after surgery, 60
anxiety, 58, 108, 110
getting counseling, 113
grieving, 107-109
see also Body image and
Relationships
Erectile dysfunction, see Men

F

Familial adenomatous polyposis
(FAP), 20-21
Fatigue, after surgery, 64
see also Sleeping
Food, see Diet and nutrition

G

Gas, reduction of, 86-87

H

Healing, mind and body, 60-61
Healthcare professionals, dealing with,
42-43
Enterostomal Therapy (ET) nurse,
57
help after surgery, 56
questions to ask, 44-48
when to contact,
WOC nurse, 56, 57, 71
see also Homeopathy
Herbal remedies, for bladder infections,
59-60
Hirschsprung's disease, 130
see also Congenital conditions and
Children and babies

Homeopathy, post-surgery, 58-60
pre-surgery, 48-50
Hospital stay, 55-57

I

Ileal conduit, *see* Conduit
Ileoanal reservoir, 32-33
Ileostomy, 30-31
diet and, 90-91
management and care of, 68-69
potassium and sodium, 90-91
types of, 31
see also Stoma, location of
Immunosuppressant drugs, 47
Inflammatory bowel disease (IBD),
21-22
diet and, 22
risk for colorectal cancer and, 22
smoking and, 22
symptoms of, 22-23
treatment for, 23-24
vitamin D deficiency, 22
Injury, 18
skin and, 77
International Ostomy Association, 53,
142
Intestinal reservoir (Koch pouch), 34-
35
Intimacy and sexuality, *See* Relationships *and* Sex and sexuality
Irrigation, 66-67
techniques, 67
travel tips, 103

J

J-pouch, *See* Appliances

K

Koch pouch, 34-35

L

Lifestyle, job and, 97-98
recovery and, 60-61

sports and activities, 72
traveling, 99-103

M

Medical professionals, *See* Healthcare
professionals
Medication, 95-96
antibiotics, 60
immunosuppressants, 47
Men and ostomies, 117-118
body image, 122
erecticle dysfunction and treatment
of, 118-121
gay men, 122
tips, 122-123

O

Odor, 74,
charcoal filters, 74
deodorant tablets, 74
deodorants, 73
diet and reduction of, 84-86
drops or sprays, 73
parsley or chlorophyll, 91
urostomy and fluid intake, 91-92
See also Diet and nutrition
Ostomy, 15-18
basic care, 47, 63-64
problems with care, 128-129
Q & A, 74-77
recognizing problems, 77
suppliers, 150-153
supplies, 47
types of, 25-29
Ostomate's rights, 53-54

P

Physocological concerns, *See* Surgery,
recovery after
Polyps, 20-21
Pregnancy and childbirth, 114-117

R

Rectum, 30, 45
Relationships, 105-112, *see also* Sex
    and sexuality
Resources and information, 141-155
Risk factors for colorectal cancer, 19

S

Seniors and ostomy care, *See* Elderly
Sex and sexuality, 105-107
    communication with partner,
        111-112
    effects of surgery on, 109-110
    intercourse after surgery, 110-111
    men and, 117-122
    nerve damage, 109-110, 112
    professional support, 107
    resources and information, 154
    smaller pouch products, 72
    tips, 122-123
    women and, 112-113
Sigmoid colostomy, 29
Skin care, 92
    causes of skin problems, 93-95
    cleaning, 92-93
    cleansers, 73
    skin barriers, 73
Sleeping, aromatherapy and, 50
    see also Fatigue
Spina bifida, 130
    see also Congenital conditions *and*
        Children and babies
Sports, 98-99
Stoma, bleeding, 77
    location of, 45-46
    plug, 68
    size and shape of, 47
Supplies and suppliers, 47, 150-153
Surgery, after, 55-56
    appliances while recovering, 71
    discontinuing immunosuppressants
        prior to, 47
    ostomate's rights, 53-54
    preparing for, 41-44
    procedures before, 52-53

questions to ask prior to, 44-48
recovery tips, 60-61
returning to work after, 97-98
smoking and, 48
surgical reversal (closure), 30
see also Colostomy, Ileostomy *and*
    Urostomy

T

Teenagers and ostomies, 134-136
Traveling, 99-103

U

Ulcerative colitis, 16,21
    resources and information, 149-150
    see also Inflammatory bowel disease
Urostomies, 37
    basic care and management of,
        69-70
    colonic conduit, 38
    diet and, 91-92
    fluid intake, 95
    ileal conduit, 37
    problems with, 95
see also Medication *and* Vitamin

V

Vitamins, vitamin C, 96
    vitamin D deficiency, 22
    see also Medications

W

Weight, 82
    changes in, 65; 76, 82
WOC nurse, *see* Healthcare
    professionals
Women and ostomies, 112-114
    body image, 113-114
    pregnancy and delivery, 114-117
    see also Relationships *and* Sex and
        sexuality
Work, 97-98

ISBN 141200081-5